A Bridge to Recovery

An Introduction to 12-Step Programs

A Bridge to Recovery

An Introduction to 12-Step Programs

Robert L. DuPont, M.D.

President, Institute for Behavior and Health, Inc.,
Rockville, Maryland, and
Clinical Professor of Psychiatry,
Georgetown University School of Medicine,
Washington, DC

and

John P. McGovern, M.D.

Clinical Professor of Medicine,
University of Texas Medical School at Houston,
and Clinical Professor of Pediatrics and Microbiology,
Baylor College of Medicine, Houston, Texas

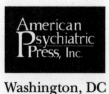

Washington, DC
London, England

Note: The authors have worked to ensure that all information in this book concerning drug dosages, schedules, and routes of administration is accurate as of the time of publication and consistent with standards set by the U.S. Food and Drug Administration and the general medical community. As medical research and practice advance, however, therapeutic standards may change. For this reason and because human and mechanical errors sometimes occur, we recommend that readers follow the advice of a physician who is directly involved in their care or the care of a member of their family.

Copyright © 1994 American Psychiatric Press, Inc.
ALL RIGHTS RESERVED
Manufactured in the United States of America on acid-free paper
97 96 95 94   4 3 2 1
First Edition

American Psychiatric Press, Inc.
1400 K Street, N.W., Washington, DC   20005

Library of Congress Cataloging-in-Publication Data
DuPont, Robert L., 1936–   .
    A bridge to recovery : an introduction to 12-step programs /
    Robert L. DuPont, and John P. McGovern. — 1st ed.
        p.   cm.
    Includes bibliographical references and index.
    ISBN 0-88048-669-4 (alk. paper)
    1. Twelve-step programs—United States.   2. Substance abuse—
Treatment.   3. Alcoholics—Rehabilitation.   4. Narcotic addicts—
Rehabilitation.   I. McGovern, John P., 1921–   .   II. Title.
RC564.73.D87   1994
362.29′186—dc20   93-26758
                                                                            CIP

British Library Cataloguing in Publication Data
A CIP record is available from the British Library.

For all addicted people
   and those who love and respect them,
With hope for lasting recovery
   that can only be achieved
Through hard work—
   One day at a time.

Contents

Preface

This book grew out of a series of intensive, prolonged discussions in early 1990 concerning the best ways people in the helping professions could integrate the 12-step programs—such as Alcoholics Anonymous and programs modeled on it—into their everyday activities. We drew three conclusions as a result of these discussions. First, we had no intent to influence in any way the 12-step programs themselves. We did not need to be convinced that these programs really work for millions of addicted people. Second, we wanted to focus on the process of referral to the 12-step programs. We were strongly interested in research into the best ways to make such referrals, or "introductions," to 12-step programs. We conceptualized our mission as helping to build bridges between major social institutions, such as health care, education, and religion, and the specific 12-step programs. Third, we wanted to bring into this process individuals with substantial experience on both sides of these bridges—those with profound knowledge of the nation's major social institutions, and those with deep roots in the 12-step programs. We were pleased that the American Psychiatric Press was interested in publishing our book, ensuring that the work would be available for many years to those in the helping professions involved in the referral process.

In the fall of 1990, to help achieve these goals, the Institute for Behavior and Health established an expert committee that met for 2 days to develop the initial plan for this book. These committee members spoke as individuals, knowledgeable of 12-step programs and/or of social institutions including health care, substance abuse treatment, education, religion, the workplace, and the criminal justice system. The committee discussed a number of topics, including the role of the 12-step fellowships in treatment, accessibility to 12-step meetings, appropriate introductory techniques, and the role of individuals and social institutions in the referral process. A research agenda was outlined addressing the characteristics of alcoholics and/or addicts who profit from 12-step meetings, determining useful referral strategies, and formulating effective research designs.

Based on the spirited and informative discussions at the meeting, a draft manuscript was written and circulated to the committee members for their comments and additions. Sarah Shiraki handled the day-to-day staff work for this project at the Institute for Behavior and Health and helped with the writing of the manuscript. The book is the result of the collaboration of everyone involved in this ambitious project, although the authors take final responsibility for its content.

This book is dedicated to promoting recovery from addiction through referral from the primary social institutions of modern life—the family, the health care system, the criminal justice system, schools, religion, and the workplace—to the 12-step programs. Our goals are to provide members of social institutions with useful information about 12-step programs and to find more effective ways to build and to use bridges to these programs. We believe that making good introductions to 12-step programs is a vital step for these social institutions if they are to fulfill their basic humanitarian missions for the many alcoholics and addicts they now serve. Valuable opportunities exist for direct involvement between the representatives of these institutions and members of 12-step fellowships. This book encourages the strengthening of connections on both sides of the bridge.

Robert L. DuPont, M.D.
John P. McGovern, M.D.

Committee Members

Robert L. DuPont, M.D., Co-Chairman
President, Institute for Behavior and Health, Inc., Rockville,
Maryland; Clinical Professor of Psychiatry, Georgetown
University School of Medicine, Washington, DC

John P. McGovern, M.D., Co-Chairman
Clinical Professor of Medicine, University of Texas Medical
School at Houston, Houston, Texas; Clinical Professor of
Pediatrics and Microbiology, Baylor College of Medicine,
Houston, Texas

Hamilton Beazley
Former President, National Council on Alcoholism and
Drug Dependence, New York, New York

Peter Bell
President, Bell and Associates, Minneapolis, Minnesota

Thomasina Borkman, Ph.D.
Professor of Sociology, Department of Sociology, George
Mason University, Fairfax, Virginia

Ronald C. Brand
Executive Director, Minnesota Association of Community,
Mental Health Programs, Inc., St. Paul, Minnesota

David Brenna, M.S.
Special Projects Manager, Division of Alcohol and Substance
Abuse, Department of Social and Health Services, Olympia,
Washington

Barry S. Brown, Ph.D.
Chief, Community Research Branch, National Institute on
Drug Abuse, Rockville, Maryland

Roger Bulger, M.D.
President, Association of Academic Health Centers,
Washington, DC

Ralph S. Carpenter
Professor of Pastoral Counseling, Albert B. Chandler Medical
Center, University of Kentucky, Lexington, Kentucky

George De Leon, Ph.D.
Director, Center for Therapeutic Community Research at National
Development and Research Institutes, Inc., New York, New York

Frances Jemmott Dory
Executive Director, California Self-Help Center, Los Angeles,
California

Richard K. Fuller, M.D.
Director, Division of Clinical Prevention and Research, National
Institute on Alcohol Abuse and Alcoholism, Rockville, Maryland

Gordon Grimm
Vice Chair, Hazelden Institute, Center City, Minnesota

Henrick Harwood
Senior Policy Analyst, Office of National Drug Control Policy,
Executive Office of the President, Washington, DC

The Honorable Harold Hughes
Chairman of the Board, Harold Hughes Centers, Des Moines,
Iowa; Chairman of the Board, Society of Americans for
Recovery, Des Moines, Iowa; Chairman of the Board, SOAR
Foundation, Des Moines, Iowa; Chairman of the Board, Hughes
Foundation, Des Moines, Iowa

John E. King, L.C.S.W.
Professor, Social Work Program, University of Arkansas,
Fayetteville, Arkansas

The Reverend William B. Lowry, Jr.
Chief, Special Projects Division, State Alcohol and Drug Abuse
Administration, Maryland Department of Health and Mental
Hygiene, Baltimore, Maryland

Ron Magers
Anchor, WMAQ/NBC Television, Chicago, Illinois

Louis J. Medvene, Ph.D.
Assistant Professor of Psychology, Wichita State University,
Wichita, Kansas

The Right Reverend Robert O. Miller
Bishop of the Episcopal Diocese of Alabama, Birmingham,
Alabama

Patricia Owen, Ph.D.
Director of Research, Hazelden Foundation, Minneapolis,
Minnesota

The Reverend Thomas Price, Ph.D.
Bowie, Maryland

Beny J. Primm, M.D.
Associate Administrator, Office of Treatment Improvement,
Rockville, Maryland; Representative from Al-Anon Family Group
Headquarters, New York, New York

Frank Riessman, Ph.D.
Director, National Self-Help Clearinghouse, Graduate School
and University Center of the City University of New York,
New York, New York

Stephen W. Ringer, B.A., C.A.P.
Public Information Chairperson, W.S.C.N.A., Miami, Florida

Gail N. Schultz, M.D.
Medical Director, Betty Ford Center, Eisenhower Medical
Center, Rancho Mirage, California

Arlene B. Seal, Ph.D.
CWD International, Inc., Drug Prevention, Education and
Counseling, Pittsburgh, Pennsylvania

Richard B. Seymour
Training and Prevention Consultant, Haight-Ashbury Free
Medical Clinics, San Francisco, California; President, Westwind
Associates, Sausalito, California

D. Dwayne Simpson, Ph.D.
Professor and Director, Institute of Behavioral Research,
Texas Christian University, Ft. Worth, Texas

James K. Stewart
Former Director, National Institute of Justice, Washington, DC

Introduction

This book explores the 12-step revolution, reviews the existing strategies used by many social institutions to harness the hope these programs provide, and offers suggestions for wider use of these linkage techniques. It provides practical suggestions and a research agenda that has the potential for answering some of the central questions about the effectiveness of referrals to 12-step programs: For whom do these programs work best? What are the best ways for social institutions to access the 12-step programs? How can the effectiveness of referrals be improved? This book addresses these questions by taking a careful look at the 12-step programs and the issues involved in making referrals that can result in the greatest benefit for the estimated one in four Americans affected by alcoholism and/or addiction to other drugs.

The modern drug abuse epidemic, which began in the mid-1960s, continues to take a tragic toll on individuals, families, and communities. Many of the social costs (particularly those related to urban violence, prison populations, and babies born of addicted mothers) continue at unprecedented levels.

More than 16% of Americans—40 million people—will experience problems of chemical dependence at some point in their lives. At any given time, approximately one-fourth of that number are actively abusing alcohol or other drugs (Regier et al. 1990). The number of alcoholics is about twice the number of people who abuse all other drugs. About three-fourths of these chemically dependent people are males. The social costs of chemical dependence exceed $114 billion a year (Rice et al. 1990).

The encouraging news is that national drug use surveys indicate a gradual reduction in illicit drug use among Americans, especially among adolescents and young adults. In recent years, rates of alcohol use also have fallen slightly for all age groups. In 1991, the percentages reporting any illicit drug use during the past year decreased from the 1990 level by 3% among high school seniors, 4% among college students, and 4% among all young adults ages 19–28 (Johnson et al. 1992). The National Household Survey reflects a similar trend among younger users. In 1979, 26% of individuals between the ages of 12 and 17 reported use of illicit drugs in the past year; by 1990, that percentage had dropped to 15.9%. Illicit drug use in the previous 12 months in people aged 18 to 25 dropped from 49.4% in 1979 to 28.7% in 1990. Individuals 26 and older showed little change in their drug use from 1979 to 1990— that percentage stood at 10% in 1979, increased to 13.3% in 1985, then dropped again to 10.1% in 1990 (National Institute on Drug Abuse [NIDA] 1991).

As encouraging as these figures are, however, the absolute numbers are still very large; and in many high-risk populations, there have been no declines in illicit drug use. For example, the percentage of booked arrestees in 24 surveyed cities has not fallen in parallel to the decreases in high school and household surveys. In addition, although alcohol use is illegal among most high school and college students, 88% of high school seniors report at least trying alcohol and 54% report alcohol use in the prior 30 days. Most worrisome are reports of heavy drinking (defined as five or more drinks in a row at least once in the prior 2-week period) among high school and college students. Using this definition of excessive drinking, 30% of high school seniors and 43% of college students report this level of alcohol use (Johnson et al. 1992).

In addition to the already tragically high costs of alcohol abuse in the United States, drug use creates an enormous chemical dependence problem. Although the news of fewer first-time and casual users of illicit drugs is encouraging, a huge problem remains with the hard-core users of these substances. Long-term users crowd jails and prisons and fill treatment centers throughout the country. This population of addicted people possesses fewer community, family, and financial resources and comes most frequently to the attention of social institutions. For these Americans, and for their friends and families, any evidence that the country may be turning the corner on drug abuse bears little resemblance to their personal experience.

Nationally, expenditures in the fight against drug abuse have skyrocketed since the 1986 death of college basketball star Len Bias, and the emergence of crack cocaine prompted a renewed national commitment to solving the problems of chemical dependence. Expenditures for enforcement of drug laws have risen most sharply.

Despite the national resolve to eradicate the illicit drug problem, controversies about American drug policies abound. The debates extend from legalizing all drugs, eliminating the profit from the illicit drug market, to creating and enforcing additional illicit drug use sanctions. Some critics of current policies propose increased funding for treatment (as opposed to law enforcement) or for prevention and education (as opposed to treatment and law enforcement). Although all agree on the importance of enforcement, prevention, and treatment, there is widespread disagreement about the relative efficacy of each of those efforts, the level of resources each should command, and the strategies each should include. Controversies about the use of drug tests in the workplace are particularly volatile. In addition, it has become common to equate the use of alcohol and tobacco with the use of illicit drugs and to ask for an evenhanded allocation of prevention and treatment resources between the licit (for adults) and illicit drugs.

Included in the economic costs to our society of alcohol and other drug use, amounting to billions of dollars, is the cost for the large number of people who enter alcohol or drug treatment each year. On September 30, 1989, there were 734,955 people in drug treatment programs in the United States (Alcohol, Drug Abuse, and Mental Health Administration [ADAMHA] 1990). Large sums of money are expended on addiction treatment programs, and considerable time is lost from families and employment.

In the 1990s, however, there is hope in the long, painful national battle against drug abuse. Against this backdrop of conflict and controversy about drug use, a quiet and powerful revolution is growing that is unrelated to the political and budgetary battles that have captured the nation's attention. This revolution is the family of 12-step programs based on Alcoholics Anonymous (AA). Alcoholics Anonymous is the source of the Twelve Steps and Twelve Traditions that are fundamental to this diverse family of recovery fellowships. Twelve-step programs are free of charge to everyone regardless of socioeconomic status. The programs neither seek nor accept public or private funding. They do not require health insurance. They are not led by professionals. Twelve-step programs do not seek the support or approval of any individual, group, or government agency. They are not licensed by any bureaucracy, nor are they affiliated with any religious group. The 12-step fellowships are not treatment programs, and they do not compete with or replace formal treatment of any kind. They are fellowships that offer a program of recovery that an individual may use either in lieu of or to complement and enhance professional treatment. The programs extend far beyond a period of relatively brief professionally run treatment of addictions, including addiction to alcohol and other drugs (also known as chemical dependence).

For millions of Americans, 12-step programs work one day at a time to change the slavery of addiction to alcohol and other drugs into the freedom of recovery. These programs appear to many to be the nation's best chance of winning the war against alcohol and drug abuse and of rebuilding stronger, healthier families and communities.

Over the past decade, the self-help or mutual-aid movement has taken on a life of its own. Bookstores carry numerous shelves of material, and clearinghouses publish multipage lists of meetings. By definition, a self-help group is one that is run without professional leadership. An individual decides to get help and support for a problem and seeks out a supportive group in which to share information and experiences and to find better ways to cope with the problem. Volunteers take care of administrative details, and there is no cost to participants.

The 12-step programs do not see themselves only as "self-help" because these programs are group efforts based on well-organized techniques. Twelve-step programs balk at being called "mutual-aid" programs because recovery also is seen as coming from a "higher power" rather than from willpower. In the AA Preamble, Alcoholics Anonymous defines itself as an organization:

> Alcoholics Anonymous is a fellowship of men and women who share their experience, strength and hope with each other that they may solve their common problem and help others to recover from alcoholism.
>
> The only requirement for membership is a desire to stop drinking. There are no dues or fees for AA membership; we are self-supporting through our own contributions. AA is not allied with any sect, denomination, politics, organization or institution; does not wish to engage in any controversy, neither endorses nor opposes any causes. Our primary purpose is to stay sober and help other alcoholics to achieve sobriety.[1]

In this book we use the words "self-help" and "mutual-aid" to describe these groups with the understanding that these words do not adequately describe these complex and unique programs. We also recognize that many of these fellowships do not use either "self-help" or "mutual-aid" in describing their programs. Nevertheless, because this book is written primarily for those who are in a position to make referrals to the 12-step programs, the words "self-help" and "mutual-aid" are used to help potential referral sources distinguish the 12-step fellowships from the professionally run mental health treatment programs for addiction to alcohol and other drugs.

Self-help clearinghouses that respond to individuals seeking help for a behavioral, relationship, or health-related problem include 12-step programs in their listings. The number of Americans now participating in self-help groups, including 12-step programs, is unclear; but recently it was estimated that there are about 15 million people attending 500,000 separate meetings in any given week (Leerhsen et al. 1990). The growth rate of the 12-step groups is estimated to be about 3% per year (Saylor et al. 1990). AA and

---

[1] Copyright © by The AA Grapevine, Inc. Reprinted with permission.

Al-Anon alone hold more group meetings than all other self-help groups combined (Leventhal et al. 1988). AA currently has more than 2 million members in more than 130 countries (Alcoholics Anonymous General Service Office, personal communication, September 1993).

The 12-step fellowships, built on Alcoholics Anonymous, provide hope and help for millions of people worldwide at more than 160,000 meetings (White and Madara 1992). The Twelve Steps have become the only response to the problem of chemical dependence that is large enough, effective enough, and diverse enough to offer real hope of ending the epidemic of alcohol and other drug abuse through the process of recovery. Twelve-step fellowships address the problems of family members of addicted people and a wide range of other behavioral problems including gambling and eating disorders. Because alcohol is the most widely used addictive substance and because Alcoholics Anonymous is the original and still the largest 12-step fellowship, many of the examples used in this book refer to AA.

This book focuses on addiction to alcohol and other drugs and on the role of the 12-step fellowships, Alcoholics Anonymous and other fellowships modeled on it, in the process of recovery from addiction. In the language of recovery, being "sober" usually refers to not using alcohol, being "clean" usually refers to not using nonmedical drugs, and being "abstinent" refers to refraining from either alcohol or nonmedical drug use.

The text uses the terms "alcoholic," "addict," and "addicted people." As used in this book, an alcoholic is a person who abuses alcohol, an addict is a person who abuses illegal drugs, and an addicted person abuses both. For many people, the terms "alcoholic" or "addict" bring to mind a down-and-out derelict panhandling passersby on the street or injecting heroin in an alley. But these terms also can refer to the highly educated professional who has a serious problem with alcohol, or the adolescent who is a heavy smoker of marijuana. Members of 12-step programs introduce themselves at meetings by saying, "Hi, my name is Joe, and I am an alcoholic," or "My name is Barbara, and I am an addict." Use of these blunt terms directly confronts the denial that is the driving force of the disease of addiction. Literature distributed by the 12-step programs uses the straightforward terms *alcoholic* and *addict*.

All of the major American social institutions are severely affected by the problems of chemical dependence. These institutions include the family, health care and drug treatment facilities, educational institutions, religious organizations, and the workplace. A top priority in the national effort to reduce the suffering caused by chemical dependence is to find methods for these institutions to identify chemical dependence and to provide access to the 12-step fellowships for help, both for those who are chemically dependent themselves and for those who are struggling to cope with chemically dependent friends, family members, and colleagues (DuPont and McGovern 1992).

The 12-step movement is not without controversy. Some critics have misgivings about the fellowships, ranging from doubts about their effectiveness to concerns about 12-step fellowships being used as an excuse to cut funding for other needed programs. Additional criticism has been voiced about the spiritual underpinnings of these programs and their acceptability for women and minority group members. Despite criticism, which seems to have increased as these programs have grown during the past decade, the Twelve Steps themselves appear to be easily grasped and readily accepted by people from varied backgrounds—laborers and professionals, people who did not complete high school and people who have postdoctoral education, the wealthy and the poor. Twelve-step fellowships offer meetings for groups with special needs, including women, youth, Hispanics, gay men and lesbians, and people with hearing impairments. In addition, the 12-step programs appear to many observers to be uniquely effective in establishing and maintaining long-term recovery from addiction and in providing lifelong help for the families of problem drinkers and drug abusers.

One of the more remarkable developments of the last decade has been that many traditional American social institutions have begun to integrate 12-step meetings into many of their basic programs, producing a newly effective response to the problems of alcohol and other drug abuse. One of the best examples of 12-step program use is private inpatient chemical dependence treatment—the so-called Minnesota model, which integrates the 12-step fellowships into the medical treatment of addiction. Today, when many Americans go to drug and alcohol treatment programs, they and their families learn about the disease of addiction and are introduced to long-term participation in the fellowships of Alcoholics Anonymous or Narcotics Anonymous (NA) and their companion programs, the Al-Anon Family Groups and Nar-Anon.

The driving while impaired (DWI) programs (known in some states as driving while intoxicated or driving under the influence [DUI]), which are concerned with drug- and alcohol-impaired drivers, also routinely use the 12-step programs. Throughout the nation, the DWI programs incorporate the recognition of alcoholism and drug addiction as diseases and encourage regular attendance at 12-step meetings.

The DWI programs and drug and alcohol treatment programs provide important models for other social institutions in using the 12-step fellowships as integral parts of their activities for virtually all participants. The criminal justice system (building on the DWI model) is using 12-step meetings in prison programs, probation, and parole. Religious institutions for decades have been the most common sites for 12-step meetings. Increasingly, 12-step fellowships are being used to address the problems of addiction among parishioners and clergy. In the workplace, employee assistance programs (EAPs) have introduced 12-step programs to millions of Americans. Student assistance programs (SAPs) are beginning to do the same for schools across the nation.

The 12-step programs are not the magic bullet in the war against drugs. They are not necessarily the best approach for everyone with an addiction, and they are not a reason to abandon other useful responses to alcohol and other drug problems. However, the 12-step programs do offer a unique resource to millions of Americans. We must now develop more effective methods for social institutions to make referrals to 12-step programs. Professionals who are not themselves experts in addiction or recovery must become familiar with referral opportunities and techniques. This book is written with that goal in mind.

A research program is needed to study the referral process and to identify effective introduction methods. No one referral technique works for everyone; more data are needed to shape more effective and more specifically tailored techniques to introduce people to the 12-step fellowships. The focus of this much-needed new research should be on the referral process and not on the 12-step programs themselves. The 12-step groups are accepted as they are; no recommendations are made to modify or adapt the organization or structure of the fellowships. This approach, focused on referral, respects the independence of the 12-step fellowships and the principles of anonymity on which they are based.

This book is organized into three sections. Section I is divided into six chapters in which we describe the Twelve Steps and Twelve Traditions of Alcoholics Anonymous and discuss the history of the 12-step movement, its philosophy, the structure of meetings, and background information. The introductory process and controversial issues for individuals and institutions making referrals to 12-step programs are also covered in Section I. In Section II, we discuss the social institutions that are involved with problems of addiction and suggests ways to tap into the full potential of the 12-step programs. In Section III, we describe current research knowledge about referrals to the 12-step programs and outline steps to increase this knowledge base. The issue of research is vital, because the full commitment of America's social institutions will occur only when the effectiveness of referral to 12-step programs is demonstrated.

Further materials are available from the individual 12-step fellowship headquarters and other resources listed in the Appendix.

SECTION I

The 12-Step Programs

- Twelve Steps of Alcoholics Anonymous
- Twelve Traditions of Alcoholics Anonymous

Addiction is slavery—slavery to behaviors and to the feelings those behaviors produce. The model for understanding addiction is alcoholism, the experience of being powerless over the urge to drink. Recovery is the process of overcoming active addiction and changing one's lifestyle to maintain abstinence.

All 12-step programs are modeled on Alcoholics Anonymous. These "fellowships," so called because of the central role of affiliation with other recovering people, are the heart of the recovery process. Twelve-step fellowships are sweeping not only the United States but the world. Although no firm data are available, mutual-aid programs, including the 12-step fellowships, are estimated to reach 15 million Americans and 5 million other addicted people and family members throughout the world, with about 50,000 meetings each week in the United States and 10,000 in the rest of the world. These numbers have multiplied fourfold in the last decade, reflecting the rapid growth of mutual-aid programs (Leerhsen et al. 1990).

1

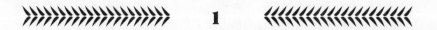

The Twelve Steps and Twelve Traditions of Alcoholics Anonymous

At the core of the 12-step fellowships are the Twelve Steps and the Twelve Traditions. Part of one or both of the documents often is read aloud in some format at 12-step meetings to help provide a basic orientation to the program.

The Twelve Steps and the Twelve Traditions were originally formulated by AA between 1935 and 1939 and first published in 1939 in *Alcoholics Anonymous* (1976), commonly known as the "Big Book." Each succeeding non-AA 12-step fellowship has adapted them to its specific needs with as few changes as possible. The Twelve Steps form a program of recovery and a blueprint for achieving personal spiritual growth. The Twelve Traditions are the bylaws and code of ethics of all the 12-step fellowships. Each point is open to some degree of interpretation—especially that of a "higher power"—but the basic program is immutable.

Although the Twelve Steps are discussed at meetings, their practice is personal and involves each member and his or her sponsor. The Twelve Traditions are guidelines governing the entire fellowship, not a vague accumulation of practices.

The Twelve Steps of Alcoholics Anonymous

1. We admitted we were powerless over alcohol—that our lives had become unmanageable.
2. Came to believe that a Power greater than ourselves could restore us to sanity.
3. Made a decision to turn our will and our lives over to the care of God *as we understood Him.*
4. Made a searching and fearless moral inventory of ourselves.
5. Admitted to God, to ourselves, and to another human being, the exact nature of our wrongs.
6. Were entirely ready to have God remove all these defects of character.
7. Humbly asked Him to remove our shortcomings.
8. Made a list of all persons we had harmed, and became willing to make amends to them all.
9. Made direct amends to such people wherever possible, except when to do so would injure them or others.
10. Continued to take personal inventory and when we were wrong promptly admitted it.
11. Sought through prayer and meditation to improve our conscious contact with God *as we understood Him,* praying only for knowledge of His will for us and the power to carry that out.
12. Having had a spiritual awakening as the result of these steps, we tried to carry this message to alcoholics and to practice these principles in all our affairs.

The first three of the Twelve Steps provide a foundation for abstinence by accepting the problem and acknowledging the hopelessness and futility of former egocentric efforts to deal with it; by coming to believe in the existence of a spiritual force that could effectively rescue the alcoholic; and by committing to a trust and reliance on this "Power greater than ourselves." The remaining nine steps outline the means of resolving the problem.

Steps Four, Five, Six, and Seven call for making a personal moral inventory, revealing the results of that inventory to God and another human being (usually one's sponsor), becoming willing to have one's character defects or shortcomings removed, and humbly asking one's Higher Power to remove them. Steps Eight and Nine involve the interpersonal sphere—making amends and restitution to others. Step Ten is a maintenance step, bringing together all of the elements from Steps Four through Nine into a daily process of awareness, self-evaluation, and making amends as indicated. Step Eleven expands one's spiritual relationship with God through prayer and meditation, and Step Twelve brings the individual full circle by continuing to practice the principles embodied in each of the steps and by helping others with alcohol and addiction problems. Only two of the steps (Steps One and Twelve) mention alcohol or addiction, whereas six of the steps mention God or the Higher Power.

The Twelve Traditions of Alcoholics Anonymous were first drawn up in an approximation of their present form in 1946. As the Twelve Steps represent the blueprint for maintaining sobriety and spiritual development of individuals within the fellowships, the Twelve Traditions represent the guiding structure or constitution of the fellowship as a whole. Professionals and others interested in working cooperatively with 12-step fellowships need an understanding of the Twelve Traditions.

The Twelve Traditions
of Alcoholics Anonymous

1. Our common welfare should come first; personal recovery depends upon AA unity.
2. For our group purpose there is but one ultimate authority— a loving God as He may express Himself in our group conscience. Our leaders are but trusted servants; they do not govern.
3. The only requirement for AA membership is a desire to stop drinking.

4. Each group should be autonomous except in matters affecting other groups or AA as a whole.
5. Each group has but one primary purpose—to carry its message to the alcoholic who still suffers.
6. An AA group ought never endorse, finance, or lend the AA name to any related facility or outside enterprise, lest problems of money, property, and prestige divert us from our primary purpose.
7. Every AA group ought to be fully self-supporting, declining outside contributions.
8. Alcoholics Anonymous should remain forever nonprofessional, but our service centers may employ special workers.
9. AA, as such, ought never be organized; but we may create service boards or committees directly responsible to those they serve.
10. Alcoholics Anonymous has no opinion on outside issues; hence the AA name ought never be drawn into public controversy.
11. Our public relations policy is based on attraction rather than promotion; we need always maintain personal anonymity at the level of press, radio, and films.
12. Anonymity is the spiritual foundation of all our traditions, ever reminding us to place principles before personalities.

The Twelve Traditions were formulated to guarantee the unity, integrity, and smooth functioning of the 12-step fellowships. Although these recovery groups are commonly known by their designation as 12-step programs, the Twelve Traditions are of no less importance. Just as the Twelve Steps to recovery are suggestions, the Twelve Traditions do not forbid anything but are phrased positively as "shoulds" and "oughts." They help maintain the integrity and smooth functioning of the fellowship. The concepts of anonymity and nonalliance are especially significant. Traditions Two, Eleven, and Twelve safeguard the fellowship against the development of overzealous, self-serving leaders who may publicly present dubious impressions of themselves or of their respective fellowships. Traditions Three and Ten refer to AA's singleness of purpose by focusing on alcohol and not on outside issues. Tradition Six illustrates the potential damage in endorsing, financing, or lending the AA name to any outside enterprise. Anonymity, as stated in Tradition Twelve, is a safeguard for individuals against negative reactions that may result from their exposure as an addict or alcoholic. Anonymity also encourages individuals in recovery to look beyond themselves to the essential premises of the Twelve Steps.

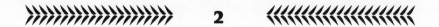

2

The Story of Addiction

- Definition of Addiction
- Disease Concept of Addiction
- Philosophy of the 12-Step Programs

Addiction and Recovery

Addiction is defined by the American Society of Addiction Medicine (1990) as a disease process characterized by the continued use of a specific psychoactive substance despite physical, psychological, or social harm. For purposes of this publication, addiction means loss of control over the use of alcohol and other drugs including marijuana and cocaine. Addiction to prescribed medicines, called "controlled substances," is also possible. (The distinctions between medical use and nonmedical use of drugs are discussed in Chapter 7.) An addicted person uses the addictive substance at times and in ways that produce progressively more serious negative consequences, including deleterious impacts on the user's health, safety, and relationships.

The disease concept of alcoholism has gained acceptance among health care professionals in recent years. To be classified as a "disease," a disorder or problem usually must have all of the following characteristics:

1. A clear biological basis;
2. Identifiable, specific characteristics;
3. Predictable progression and outcome; and
4. Absence of volitional control.

A comprehensive review published in two issues of *Psychiatric Annals* entitled "The Disease Concept of Alcoholism and Drug Addiction," edited by psychiatrist Norman S. Miller, concluded that alcoholism met all of the criteria for a disease (Miller 1991a, 1991b; Miller and Chappel 1991). David Lewis, a physician specializing in internal medicine, writing in this same group of articles, concluded that, as with many other diseases, there were important psychological and social dimensions to the prevalence, course, and presentation of the disease of addiction to alcohol and other drugs (Lewis 1991). This view has become widely if not yet universally accepted in the medical and scientific communities.

In 1992, a definition of alcoholism appeared in the *Journal of the American Medical Association*. This definition was developed over a 2-year period by a 23-member expert committee of the American Society of Addiction Medicine (ASAM) and the National Council on Alcoholism and Drug Dependence. The committee sought a definition that was scientifically valid, clinically useful, and understandable by the general public. This new definition represents the mainstream medical view on the subject today:

> Alcoholism is a primary, chronic disease with genetic, psychosocial, and environmental factors influencing its development and manifestations. The disease is often progressive and fatal. It is characterized by impaired control over drinking, preoccupation with the drug alcohol, use of alcohol despite adverse consequences, and distortions in thinking, most notably denial. Each of these symptoms may be continuous or periodic. (Morse and Flavin 1992, p. 1013)

This definition can be extended to other drugs of abuse by adding the words "and other drugs" after the word "alcohol," as follows: "Addiction to alcohol and other drugs (or chemical dependence) is a primary, chronic disease with genetic, psychosocial,

and environmental factors influencing its development and manifestations. . . . "

A unique phenomenon of addictive disease is called *denial*—
the common and profound inability of the addicted person to
comprehend and accept the disease. It is as though the disease tells
addicted people that they don't have it. Addicted people deny
their use of alcohol and other drugs to themselves and to others.
Family members and others who relate to addicted people often
deny their roles in maintaining the addictive behavior. Denial is
one of the two central problems that individuals, families, and
communities need to overcome to help alleviate the problem of
addiction. The other central problem is knowing how to proceed
once the addiction is recognized. In this sense, a "cure" for addiction requires both knowing what is wrong *and* knowing what to do
about it.

Addiction is a progressive disease. If ignored, it will grow worse;
it is not self-limiting. One of the goals of social policy is to encourage earlier identification of the disease and to intervene to end the
active addiction. Once a person is addicted, the disease lasts for a
lifetime. Addicts are not responsible for their addiction, but they
are responsible for what they do with their disease and for their
own behavior (Alcoholics Anonymous 1984; DuPont 1989). There
are dissenters to the position that alcoholism and other addictions
are diseases. Stanton Peele, in his book *Diseasing of America* (1989),
argues that the disease concept of addiction offers an excuse to
alcoholics and addicts for their irresponsible behavior. Peele considers the familial pattern of addiction secondary to social and cultural factors. He states that medical treatment of addiction is no
more effective than expecting the individual to accept responsibility for behavior, and he considers most of the 12-step principles to
be unsubstantiated by research or experience. In addition, he
supports the controversial view that alcoholics can successfully
confront their problem drinking and return to controlled and rea-
sonable use of alcohol (Peele 1989, 1991).

The 12-step program fellowships are based on an enormous
body of collective experience that has been gained at tremendous

personal effort. They support the view that identifying alcoholism or addiction as a disease overcomes the guilt and shame of the drinking or drug problem and frees the individual to concentrate on those steps in the program designed to remove the destructive addictive behavior. Admitting loss of control over alcohol and other drug use is the first step in overcoming the denial that allows an addiction to maintain control over the individual's behavior (Alcoholics Anonymous 1984; Khantzian and Mack 1989; Kurtz 1987; Robertson 1988).

Twelve-step programs promote a life-style of recovery. Recovery means living drug- and alcohol-free, gaining healthy self-esteem, and maintaining sound relationships with family and community.

Foundations of the 12-Step Programs

The unique and primary aspect of each of the 12-step programs is that all members (and groups) are encouraged and motivated to "work the steps." The Twelve Steps, initiated by AA, are at the very core; indeed they are the *program* itself. They are the ingredient that sets the 12-step fellowships apart from all other self-help, mutual-aid, group therapy methodologies. The steps incorporate a pragmatic and coherent pathway leading toward a more spiritual way of life, neither encouraging nor discouraging affiliation with any particular religious sect.

Group dynamics play an important role in all mutual-aid or self-help programs, and also in the dynamics of the 12-step programs. These programs depend on an honest human connection and cooperation among members. They are coordinated and led by laypeople (fellow individuals in recovery in the 12-step programs) rather than professionals. Mutual-aid groups provide emotional support to counter isolation and an opportunity to learn from emotional pain. Twelve-step programs help people attain positive social integration and relief from self-destructive behavior through interaction with others who can empathize and identify with the participant. Group process has been found to be the best way for dealing with disaffected individuals by promoting appropriate social norms over time (Levoy 1989; Powell 1987).

The Twelve Steps offer individuals who share common self-destructive behaviors a set of practical guidelines for healthy change. Newcomers are made to feel welcome and are encouraged to return, giving a sense of belonging to an individual who may be experiencing intense alienation in other facets of life. Though many meetings are held in the morning and at noon, most meetings are held in the evening after working hours, providing an organized and predictable activity during a time of day when substance abusers are most prone to temptation and relapse. Use of positive reinforcement and supportive attention by fellow group members enhances the socialization of group members to prosocial cultural norms. Confessing a readiness to accept help is an important part of the 12-step philosophy. Acceptance is also a vital component of group interactions of mutual-aid groups. Discussing one's use of alcohol and drugs can take place in a secure, supportive, and accepting environment.

The promise of anonymity in all 12-step fellowships makes a trusting relationship possible, even with total strangers. Mutual support and a feeling of inclusion is enhanced by the commonality of experience. The giving of support is balanced by the expectation of reciprocal support. Stress reduction is another benefit of being involved in a supportive group environment. Abstinence is often stressful, as an ever-present remedy is the very substance being avoided (Wasserman and Danforth 1988).

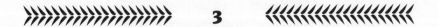

3

Development of the 12-Step Programs

- History of Alcoholics Anonymous
- Formation of Narcotics Anonymous
- Other Drug-Specific Fellowships
- Twelve-Step Family Groups
- Adult Children of Alcoholics
- Co-Dependents Anonymous
- A Guide to Selected 12-Step Fellowships

The Beginnings of Alcoholics Anonymous (AA)

In early May 1935, just 2 years after the repeal of Prohibition, Bill Wilson, an unemployed New York stockbroker with a long history of alcohol abuse, was able to stop drinking through working with practicing alcoholics. While pursuing a business opportunity in Akron, Ohio, he found himself alone, vulnerable, and in fear of taking a drink. The possibility of reverting to his former dissolute life-style distressed him. He called a local minister to get the name of another alcoholic to contact. The minister gave him the name of Henrietta Seiberling, an active member of Akron's Oxford Group, who could put him in touch with an alcoholic. The Oxford Group was a spiritual fellowship that sought to recapture the values of first-century Christianity through a program of personal self-development. Founded by Frank N. O. Buchman, a Lutheran minister from Allentown, Pennsylvania, in 1921, the Oxford Group spread widely in the 1920s and 1930s, spawning not only Alcoholics Anonymous but also today's Moral Re-Armament (MRA) (Kurtz 1987; Robertson 1988). Bill Wilson (who became known through AA as Bill W.) had been introduced to the Oxford Group in New York in November 1934 by Ebby T., a friend who achieved temporary sobriety there and later became sober in AA.

Through Henrietta Seiberling, Bill Wilson met Bob Smith, a surgeon who was an active alcoholic. Dr. Smith had been trying to stop drinking without success. On June 10, 1935, their work together culminated in the foundation of what is now known as Alcoholics Anonymous. Some of the religious precepts of the Oxford Group had an obvious influence on Bill W.'s formulation of AA philosophy, according to the book *Dr. Bob and the Good Oldtimers* (Alcoholics Anonymous 1980). For instance, the basis of the Oxford Group was the "four absolutes": absolute honesty, absolute unselfishness, absolute purity, and absolute love. According to Dr. Bob, these absolutes formed "the only yardsticks" that AA had before formulation of the Twelve Steps. The Oxford Group also had five "C"s: confidence, confession, conviction, conversion, and continuance. The group's five procedures were as follows: Give in to God; listen to God's direction; check guidance; make restitution; and share (Alcoholics Anonymous 1980).

Bill and Bob soon discovered that alcoholics did not respond well to absolutes or to the membership requirements of the Oxford Group. By 1939, AA had essentially dissolved its connections to the Oxford Group and had begun to develop its own identity. Two additional AA groups had been established in Cleveland and New York. The "Big Book" (1976), which incorporated the AA principles and practices, was completed and published in 1939 (Alcoholics Anonymous 1984; Kurtz 1987; Robertson 1988).

In 1950, AA had 90,000 members in 3,000 groups worldwide. In 1993, the membership of AA was estimated to be 89,000 groups with more than 2 million members in more than 130 countries. AA conducted a survey of members in 1992 that revealed that 65% of the membership was male, the average age of members was 42, and the average member attended 2½ meetings per week. The average length of sobriety of all AA members was 5 years, with 35% reporting more than 5 years of sobriety, 34% reporting between 1 and 5 years of sobriety, and 31% reporting less than 1 year of sobriety. The survey asked how members had been introduced to AA. (Percentages cited total more than 100%, because some respondents could name more than one referral source.) Members of AA introduced 34% to the 12-step programs, 27% were referred by a treatment program, and 29% found the groups on their own. Family members suggested AA to 21% of those surveyed, and 9% were introduced to the program by a counseling agency. The other referral sources named were physicians, 7%; employers or fellow workers, 6%; non-AA members who were friends or neighbors, 4%; Al-Anon or Alateen members, 4%; newspaper/magazine/radio/TV, 2%; and AA literature, 3% (Alcoholics Anonymous 1993).

The Development of
Narcotics Anonymous (NA)

The first Narcotics Anonymous meeting was held in the Los Angeles area in 1953. Growth of the fellowship was slow at first but accelerated in the early 1980s with the publication of NA's Basic Text in 1982. The fifth edition of *Narcotics Anonymous* was published in 1988. As of January 1988, there were more than 12,000 NA meetings in 43 countries. At that time, the fellowship was growing at a rate of 50% annually (Narcotics Anonymous 1989). In January 1993, NA reported that 26,000 groups were holding meetings in 64 countries worldwide and estimated that NA membership was doubling every 18 months (C. Prescott, personal communication, August 1993).

Narcotics Anonymous was started by individuals addicted to drugs other than alcohol who sought recovery but who found that AA did not fully meet their needs. Of the five founding members of NA, three were members of AA (Nurco and Makofsky 1981). The NA fellowship developed a broader program recognizing other compulsive activities and self-destructive mechanisms as contributing factors to addiction and accepting multiple addictions. Young addicts are often drawn to NA meetings because of the relative lack of slogans, the attention to the extended family, and the NA program's attempts to remain current with drug use trends and treatment innovations.

In adapting the Twelve Steps to their needs, the only change NA members made was the substitution of the words "our addiction" for "alcohol" in the First Step and "addicts" for "alcoholics" in the Twelfth Step to show that NA dealt with the disease of addiction rather than with any specific drug. To the question "Who are members of Narcotics Anonymous?", NA answers "Anyone who wants to stop using drugs. . . . Membership is not limited to addicts using any particular drug. . . . Recovery in NA focuses on the problem of addiction, not on any particular drug" (Narcotics Anonymous 1991, p. 1).

NA meetings follow similar formats to their AA counterparts. NA's open meetings appear to be more structured than AA's and more oriented toward educating the newcomer about NA's history, principles, and operation. All people are welcome, provided they commit to stop using drugs.

In 1989, Narcotics Anonymous conducted a survey of its membership and received more than 5,000 responses. Based on that survey, the membership of NA tends to be younger than that of AA, with 11% under age 20, 37% ages 20 to 30, 48% ages 30 to 45, and 4% over 45. Of these, 64% are men and 36% women. Forty-one percent have been abstinent for 1 to 5 years, and 7% have been abstinent for more than 5 years. Half of the respondents attend at least four meetings a week (Narcotics Anonymous 1991).

In addition to these statistics, interviews conducted by a research team in the Baltimore–Washington, DC, area found that most NA participants were addicted to more than one substance. Demographically, NA meetings tend to reflect the surrounding community in terms of race, educational level, and occupation. Membership involves honesty and a willingness to work toward recovery, rather than immediate abstinence from all drug use. Only disruptive behavior at meetings is forbidden, but the disruptive individual is urged to return to NA meetings (Nurco et al. 1983).

Members of Narcotics Anonymous undertake more direct recruitment activities than many other 12-step groups. Individual members volunteer to recruit graduates of treatment programs; to contact the criminal justice system release programs; to educate members of the clergy; and to recruit among street addicts (Nurco and Makofsky 1981).

Other Fellowships

In recent years, and usually in urban centers, several sub-fellowships based on the Twelve Steps of AA and NA have centered on specific drugs. Two organizations based on the Twelve Steps include Cocaine Anonymous (CA) and Marijuana Anonymous (MA). Generally, the members of these fellowships also attend AA and/or NA meetings but feel that specific aspects of their particular addictions are not addressed in the general meetings of the larger fellowships.

In addition to the groups centered on specific drug use, groups have been created to meet the individualized needs of women (reflected in the group Women for Sobriety) and other groups of people with special needs, such as adolescents and elderly people. Participation in these groups is usually in conjunction with attendance at regular 12-step meetings. Women for Sobriety was formed to address the unique needs of female alcoholics—needs that some women thought were not met by AA. Women helped by this alternative organization often initially attend Women for Sobriety meetings and later begin to attend AA meetings as well. The interplay between the effectiveness of the 12-step fellowships and the special needs of women alcoholics has resulted in a dual focus on the traditional and the innovative (Kirkpatrick 1986).

Other groups based on the Twelve Steps include Drugs Anonymous and Nicotine Anonymous, for individuals who want to help themselves and others recover from chemical addiction and nicotine addiction, respectively (White and Madara 1992).

Twelve-Step Family Groups

In its literature, Al-Anon Family Groups describes itself as a self-help fellowship offering a program of recovery for relatives and friends of alcoholics based on the Twelve Steps and Twelve Traditions of Alcoholics Anonymous. Alateen is a part of Al-Anon for younger family members who have been affected by someone else's drinking (Al-Anon 1989, 1990; Robertson 1988).

Al-Anon began as a natural outgrowth of AA called the Family Group. Little is known about the first meeting, but the precedent apparently was set by the wives of the founders of AA. They realized that families of AA members needed the Twelve Steps as a means of restoring normalcy to their own and to their families' lives (Al-Anon 1990; Robertson 1988). In 1954, Al-Anon incorporated as a separate worldwide fellowship known as Al-Anon Family Group Headquarters, Inc., not affiliated with AA or with any other organization.

The development of these family groups was based on the premise (only now being recognized in the treatment community) that alcoholism and other forms of addiction are family diseases. Experience indicates that nonalcoholic family members are as powerless over alcohol as their alcoholic parents, children, and spouses. Often, after the initial euphoria over an alcoholic relative's decision to seek abstinence and recovery, family members discover that emotional turmoil and shame continue. Spouses may become resentful of time spent by the alcoholic in AA meetings and activities or may find that life at home continues to deteriorate (Al-Anon 1969).

Although some people (generally family members in great emotional pain) initially may come to meetings to find out how to sober up an alcoholic or how to keep a sober alcoholic happy, Al-Anon is a support group for family members and close friends of alcoholics to focus on themselves and to improve their own lives. The message of family groups is that even if the alcoholic relative has not achieved abstinence and recovery, family members can correct the way they react to the problems of living with alcoholism and develop a better way of life through Al-Anon.

Alateen, a part of Al-Anon, was established in 1957 specifically for adolescent Al-Anon members to share experiences, learn coping strategies, and offer encouragement to one another. Their literature describes Alateen as a fellowship of teenagers whose lives have been affected by family members' drinking. Each Alateen group has an adult sponsor who is a member of Al-Anon. The sponsor is an active participant in the Alateen meeting who provides guidance and knowledge about the disease of alcoholism and about the Twelve Steps and Twelve Traditions. These groups often meet at the same time and location as Al-Anon and AA meetings to facilitate participation of family members. Members are guided toward awareness that they are not the cause of a loved one's alcoholism or addictive behaviors and that they cannot change or control anyone but themselves. The hope is that by developing their own spiritual and intellectual resources, these teenagers can develop a satisfying personal life despite alcohol-related family problems.

Of all the 12-step fellowships, Al-Anon/Alateen has the most detailed statistics available. According to the *1990 Al-Anon/Alateen Membership Survey* (Al-Anon 1991), there are more than 30,000 Al-Anon and Alateen groups worldwide. Al-Anon's membership is predominantly white (95%), female (87%), and married (male—53%, female—65%), with age distributed throughout adulthood. On the average, Al-Anon members have relationships with at least two alcoholics. Of these, 69% are spouses or former spouses, 34%

are children, 20% are parents, and 15% are siblings.

Alateen membership is slightly less homogeneous. Ethnic representation in the United States and Canada is 84% white, 5% black, 5% Hispanic, and 6% other, and the gender balance is 60% female and 40% male. The school-level composition is 21% elementary, 37% junior high, 36% senior high, 2% college, and 5% not in school. The referral source for Alateen is 58% from parents, 7% from other relatives, 18% from friends, and 10% from teachers or counselors. Members attend an average of 1.1 meetings per week; 11% of meetings are held in schools, and 2% are held in institutions.

Statistics reveal that the proportion of nonwhite members has increased from 9% to 16% since 1987, with membership increasing in both urban and rural areas. The proportion of younger Alateen members is increasing: 24% were under age 13 in 1987 compared with 31% in 1990. Referrals from teachers and counselors increased from 4% to 10% during that time, and attendance at school groups increased from 1% to 11%.

Other family mutual-aid groups based on the Twelve Steps include Nar-Anon and Families Anonymous.

Adult Children of Alcoholics and Co-Dependents Anonymous

A recent phenomenon in recovery is the growing sensitivity toward adult children of alcoholics (ACOAs). Many adults who grew up in households affected by an alcoholic family member did not have access to the burgeoning Al-Anon Family Groups. A child's fear of discovery, shame of a parent's alcoholic behavior, and inability to talk to anyone about addiction in the family frequently result in an adult unable to establish appropriate relationships. In the language of addiction, this denial is described as living with "an elephant in the living room" about which no one speaks. The family does its best to behave normally and to say nothing about the elephant, even though the elephant, which is often on a rampage, affects every move the family makes. Children who were confused and fearful of the dysfunctional family dynamics fostered by alcoholism or addiction become adults without resolving those conflicts. (See Chapter 9 for more about the dysfunctional family.) Learning that adverse childhood experiences were shared by others growing up in similar households and understanding the coping mechanisms employed to survive in such turmoil becomes a revelation to many adult children of alcoholics (DuPont and McGovern 1991b).

Within the past decade, a number of self-help organizations have emerged to provide education and support to ACOAs. Books on the subject clearly have struck a responsive chord. *Adult Children of Alcoholics,* written by Janet Woititz (1990), has sold 700,000 copies to date and was on *The New York Times* bestseller list for 45 weeks in 1987. Through books such as this, many adults are learning for the first time about the roles taken on by children in an alcoholic family (Cermak 1990; Robertson 1988). Many are seeking counseling and self-help groups to address long-neglected issues. Since the early 1980s, more than 1,500 Al-Anon Adult Children of Alcoholics groups have formed in the United States. These groups follow the same Twelve Steps and Twelve Traditions as other Al-Anon groups; however, the focus is on recovery from painful childhood experiences related to parental alcoholism (Al-Anon 1983). There is also an Adult Children of Alcoholics (ACA) group headquartered in California that has modified the Twelve Steps and Twelve Traditions of AA to address the needs of their fellowship. ACA, founded in 1976, currently holds more than 1,800 group meetings internationally (White and Madara 1992).

A recent and related movement has been the growth of Co-Dependents Anonymous. Co-dependency traces its source to early childhood and the influence of being raised by alcoholic, addicted, or otherwise dysfunctional parents. Co-dependence was defined at the First National Conference on Co-dependency in Scottsdale, Arizona, in 1989 as "a pattern of painful dependency upon compulsive behaviors and on approval from others in a search for safety, self-worth, and identity. Recovery is possible"

Table 1.   A guide to selected 12-step fellowships

Name	Abbreviation	Orientation	Number of groups
Alcoholics Anonymous	AA	Personal alcoholism	94,000
Narcotics Anonymous	NA	Personal drug addiction	22,000
Cocaine Anonymous	CA	Personal cocaine addiction	1,500
Al-Anon Family Groups	Al-Anon	Family alcoholism	32,000+
Alateen		Young Al-Anon members	4,100+
Adult Children of Alcoholics	ACA, ACOA	Adult children from alcoholic families	1,800+

Source.   White and Madara 1992.

(McGovern and DuPont 1992, p. 7). Typically, an individual becomes co-dependent by adapting to a relationship with an alcoholic or addicted parent or spouse (DuPont and McGovern 1991a; Heath and Stanton 1991). Although co-dependence was originally viewed as characterizing family members in their relationship with an alcoholic or addict, it has taken on a broader application to include other dysfunctional behavior.

Co-Dependents Anonymous was founded in 1986, adapting the Twelve Steps of Alcoholics Anonymous for men and women from dysfunctional families to help them maintain healthy adult relationships. An organization has also been formed for co-dependent members of the helping professions (White and Madara 1992).

Information on several 12-step fellowships is included in Table 1.

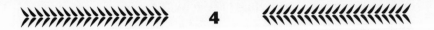

4

Notable Features of 12-Step Fellowships

- Unique Characteristics of 12-Step Programs
- The Serenity Prayer
- Types of 12-Step Meetings
- Meeting Formats
- Twelve-Step Literature

Organizational Features of 12-Step Groups

Twelve-step fellowships are distinguished by a number of unique features. They have no formal membership or application process and no dues or membership fees. The only money collected is a voluntary donation from members to cover expenses such as room rental and coffee for the meetings; no outside funds are accepted. Most groups do not keep membership records. Although the organizational characteristics vary somewhat among the 12-step fellowships, most of them share basic and rather remarkable features. For instance, AA, NA, and Al-Anon have no national presidents, officers, or hierarchies. Most centralized staff members rotate jobs in AA's General Service Office and NA's and Al-Anon's World Service Offices. These groups do not own property; the centralized service offices lease space for their staff.

No mechanism exists for disciplining or expelling a member of AA or NA who breaks one of the Twelve Traditions. Members of each organization are responsible for their own behavior.

None of the major 12-step organizations—AA, NA, or Al-Anon—accepts money from nonmembers. Members themselves are limited to a modest lifetime amount for donations. Even significant amounts of money in the form of bequests are politely declined.

Structural Features of 12-Step Meetings

Individuals become affiliated with a particular fellowship group by attending meetings regularly. Although there tends to be a core group of individuals who make up a specific, regularly scheduled meeting, other participants attend if the meeting time, place, or availability fits their needs. Members typically have one meeting that they are particularly committed to, called their "home group." Volunteer jobs are generally confined to the home group, although regular attendance may be maintained at several meetings.

The composition of meetings frequently depends on group identity, location, and population density. In rural areas, where there is a smaller and less transient population, membership attendance at meetings is relatively constant. Urban and high-density suburban areas may offer a number of meetings to a comparatively mobile fellowship population. In some instances, the constituency of a meeting may vary dramatically from week to week.

A 12-step meeting is usually held once a week at the same time and place. Meetings usually last 1 hour. They may be held at all times of the day, from early morning to late at night, with the most common meeting times being noon and 8:30 P.M. Meetings are held every day of the year. Often newer members go to more than one meeting a day, especially when they perceive a greater need for support on the advice of their sponsor (DuPont 1989). At meetings, there is an opportunity to contribute modest voluntary donations to cover expenses. Elected or appointed volunteers fill leadership functions at the meetings. These functions are usually rotated every 1 to 6 months, providing an opportunity for members to enhance their own recovery by helping others.

At a typical 12-step meeting, the secretary chooses a leader for the meeting who introduces him- or herself as an alcoholic or addict, welcomes everyone to the meeting, and invites visitors and newcomers to introduce themselves by first names only, "so that we can get to know you and talk to you after the meeting." Leaders usually are changed each meeting. During the first part of almost all meetings, members observe a moment of silence and then in unison recite the Serenity Prayer.

The Serenity Prayer

God grant me the serenity
To accept the things I cannot change;
Courage to change the things I can;
And wisdom to know the difference.[1]

Right after the Serenity Prayer, an individual member (usually called on by the meeting's leader) reads aloud a selected message from a 12-step publication—most often from the "Big Book" (1976), depending on the fellowship. General announcements typically take place either at a break midway through the meeting or at the meeting's conclusion. Many groups have a "chips system"

---

[1] These are the first four lines of a prayer generally attributed to Reinhold Niebuhr, who used it in 1943 during a service in the Congregational Church of Heath, Massachusetts, where he spent many summers. The prayer was first printed in a monthly bulletin of the Federal Council of Churches.

that may vary in its structuring from area to area, both within the United States and internationally. At these meetings, chips usually are presented just before or after the announcements.

Chips, most often in the shape of a poker chip, are tokens of accomplishment in terms of the length of sobriety. They are ceremoniously given out by the leader at most fellowship meetings to acknowledge a group member's period of abstinence, accompanied by general applause and encouragement. The more commonly acknowledged intervals during the first year of recovery are 30 days, 60 days, 90 days, 6 months, and 9 months. Thereafter, chips are bestowed on an annual basis, often at birthday meetings (see Formats of Meetings section in this chapter). The important "desire chip" (or 24-hour chip) representing an avowed desire by a newcomer to stop drinking, is given at many meetings. This is thought of as the entrance chip to AA. Similar chips often are offered by other 12-step fellowships. A desire chip also may be taken by a member who has relapsed into drinking and who wants to start anew in the program.

Meetings end when the leader asks for the usual closing, with everyone standing in a circle, holding hands, and observing a moment of silence—then reciting the Lord's Prayer, the Serenity Prayer, or whatever closing the individual fellowship group has decided on. As the group disbands, the reminders "Keep coming back!" and "It works!" are often called out.

Types of Meetings

Twelve-step meetings are divided into two primary types, open meetings and closed meetings, each having its own function within the fellowship (Alcoholics Anonymous 1993d).

Open meetings.   These meetings welcome any interested person. Twelve-step fellowships recognize that visitors may be motivated to attend an open meeting for a number of reasons. Individuals may feel a need to explore a personal drinking or drug problem, may be concerned about a friend or family member, or may simply be interested in learning about the 12-step process. All are welcome at open meetings. The only obligation placed on attendance is that of honoring the anonymity of others by not disclosing names outside of the meeting.

Closed meetings.   Depending on the specific fellowship involved, these meetings may be limited to alcoholics or addicts, those affected by another's drinking or drug use, or those who think they have a drinking or drug use problem. Closed meetings more surely safeguard members' anonymity and provide a more secure forum for the discussion of problems best understood by fellow members of a specific fellowship. The meetings are usually informal and encourage participation in the discussion. Newcomers and those who may be concerned about their anonymity within the community often find closed meetings particularly helpful.

Groups composed only of individuals with similar interests or backgrounds, such as health professionals, usually opt for a closed meeting format. By holding closed meetings, professionals can more freely discuss issues that would not be appropriate in a diverse group and can avoid encountering problems with doctor-patient or attorney-client relationships that might occur at open meetings. A number of professional self-help groups have been established in recent years, such as International Doctors in Alcoholics Anonymous (National Institute on Alcohol Abuse and Alcoholism 1986).

Formats of Meetings

Within the two types of 12-step meetings, there are several basic formats that meetings can take, although there are many variations in different areas of the United States and abroad. The following paragraphs briefly describe several common meeting formats.

Discussion meetings.   These are the most common type of AA meetings, with other 12-step fellowships usually following a similar

format. A member (frequently chosen by the secretary) presides at
a discussion meeting, opening with a topic involving recovery or
asking for a volunteer to supply one. Recurring themes include
problems in maintaining abstinence; relationships; resentments;
spirituality; and dealing with fear, anger, and anxiety. Attendees
are encouraged to participate in turn by sharing their experience,
strength, and hope according to the subject matter, but are dis-
couraged from engaging in "cross-talk" (that is, individual ex-
changes between two or more members). Supportive feelings of
openness, honesty, acceptance, goodwill, humor, patience, and
love create a deep bond among the members at these meetings.
Supportive comments from other members of the fellowship reinforce the contributions of participants.

Speaker or speaker-discussion meetings.   At these meetings,
a member of the fellowship who is chosen by the secretary (usually
well in advance of the meeting) is asked to tell his or her story at
the meeting. Although the speaker may talk for the entire meeting,
many times a speaker's presentation will be limited to 20 to 30 min-
utes, followed by a discussion of a topic chosen by the speaker or a
volunteer. When scheduling speakers, the secretary tries to achieve
a balance between regular members of a given group and visiting
members from other groups.

The speakers' presentations generally consist of a personal discussion of what their lives were like when they were dominated by
active addictive disease, their introduction to the 12-step program,
and the changes they have experienced through involvement in
the fellowship: "what it was like, what happened, and what it is like
now." At the "shorter" speaker's meetings, a speaker frequently will
suggest a topic and act as the leader for the discussion portion of
the meeting.

The first time a member tells his or her story at a meeting is an
important personal occasion marking a passage within the fellowship. Although a new speaker may find the experience difficult, it
is nearly always a positive growth experience and a valuable aid in
the process of recovery.

Step meetings.   These meetings, which incorporate the Twelve Steps, provide a blueprint for developing individual spiritual growth within the fellowship. When a regularly scheduled step meeting is initiated, it usually begins by reading and discussing Step One at the first session in a selected discussion format and focusing on a step at a time through Step Twelve at subsequent meetings. Then the group returns to Step One. Some meetings, in like fashion, elect to work their way through the Twelve Traditions as well.

Book meetings.   These meetings are similar to step meetings but involve initial readings from AA's "Big Book" ([1976] by far the most common), or other fellowship publications, such as *Living Sober: Some Methods AA Members Have Used for Not Drinking* (Alcoholics Anonymous 1975) or *Came to Believe . . . : The Spiritual Adventure of AA as Experienced by Individual Members* (Alcoholics Anonymous 1973). Those attending the meeting read and discuss passages from these publications.

Birthday meetings.   These meetings celebrate the yearly length of a member's abstinence since his or her entry into the fellowship. A group's birthday meetings usually are held monthly, marking members' durations of abstinence. The first birthday for a member celebrates 1 year of abstinence. Subsequent birthdays celebrate each additional year of sobriety.

Other meeting formats.   Some meetings adopt one particular format, which may be reflected in the meeting name, such as "12 and 12 Study," "Big Book Study," "Speaker's Meeting," or "Grapevine Discussion." Meetings may vary their format by holding 3 weeks of speaker-discussion meetings, then one step study meeting, or a similar combination. There are no established rules on meeting format, and meetings vary among fellowships, regions, and groups.

Typical 12-step meeting locations include community centers, church halls, schools, and club rooms. Meetings also may be held in institutions such as health centers, hospitals, social service agencies, drug and alcohol treatment centers, and correctional facilities.

An information number for AA can be found in the phone book of nearly every community with a 12-step fellowship. Volunteers provide meeting times and locations. "On call" fellowship members respond to personal requests for help as part of their own Twelfth Step commitment. Urban areas with numerous meetings publish a directory (frequently called "Where and When" by members) with meeting information classified by location, day of the week, time of day, and type of meeting. These directories are often available at large meetings or by calling the local central office number.

The Role of Literature and Media in 12-Step Programs

Although the 12-step fellowships do not seek or encourage publicity, an extensive variety of literature is available through the world headquarters and is provided at most local meetings. Alcoholics Anonymous offers a vast array of books and pamphlets. Introductory copies and copies for prisons and similar institutions are distributed free of charge, but other recipients (such as AA groups and treatment programs) purchase them. The pamphlets and books are sold for little more than the publishing cost.

The book *Alcoholics Anonymous* was published in 1939 and has been revised twice, the latest revision taking place in 1976. The first edition, with a large format and printed on extra-thick paper, soon became known as the "Big Book," a nickname that has endured through subsequent editions to the present. The latest edition is 575 pages long and costs about $6.00. In 1986, a softcover version was published.

Literature published by the 12-step national organizations is written primarily for the addicted person entering and sustaining recovery, or for the family member or friend of the alcoholic or addict. However, many of the pamphlets address programs, professionals, and agencies that refer individuals to the 12-step programs. The pamphlets present information to individuals unfamiliar with the Twelve Steps who interact with and advise those who experience problems with alcoholism and addiction. These titles include "Members of the Clergy Ask About Alcoholics Anonymous" (1992c), "AA as a Resource for the Health Care Professional" (1993b), "AA in Correctional Facilities" (1990c), and "AA in Treatment Facilities" (1992b). Similar topics are available from the other 12-step fellowships. Copies of these materials are available through the General Service Office listed in the Appendix.

Alcoholics Anonymous publishes a monthly journal, *The AA Grapevine,* that contains articles of interest to the community of people in recovery. The current circulation is 133,000 copies a month in 80 countries around the world (Alcoholics Anonymous 1990–1991). In an effort to make recovery available to as many people as possible, AA also edits a bimonthly newsletter called "Loners-Internationalists Meeting." This publication is mailed to 2,500 subscribers who are shut-ins or on ships at sea, unable to attend meetings in person (Robertson 1988).

The Al-Anon Family Group Headquarters publishes books and pamphlets and audiovisual materials about recovering from the family disease of alcoholism. The books include *Al-Anon Faces Alcoholism* (1990a), *Al-Anon Family Groups* (1984), *Alateen—Hope for Children of Alcoholics* (1989), . . . *In All Our Affairs* (1990b), *One Day at a Time in Al-Anon* ([1985] the most widely used volume of all, known as "ODAT" to Al-Anon members), and a recently published daily reader, *Courage to Change* (1992).

In recent years, the general public has shown increased interest in healthier life-styles, reflected in a proliferation of self-help groups (Leerhsen et al. 1990) and a related burgeoning of literature focused on self-improvement. Major publishing houses are printing books based on the 12-step themes of spirituality, meditation, and recovery, and commercial bookstores are stocking sections with recovery literature. In larger urban areas, there are stores that devote their entire stock to books, tapes, and other in-spirational materials related to 12-step recovery.

Three recently published books illustrate the type of material that is increasingly available. *The Twelve-Step Facilitation Handbook* (1992) by Joseph Nowinski and Stuart Baker offers a systematic approach to the 12-step programs for treatment and health care professionals. *The Recovery Book* (1992), written by Al J. Mooney, M.D., Arlene Eisenberg, and Howard Eisenberg, provides practical information about 12-step fellowships to recovering alcoholics and addicts. Ernest Kurtz and Katherine Ketcham have written a book, *The Spirituality of Imperfection: Modern Wisdom From Classic Stories* (1992), that captures the spiritual journey of those who embrace 12-step programs through the use of philosophical stories and per-ceptive insight.

Twelve-step programs have entered the computer age. Meet-ings of Alcoholics Anonymous are accessible via modem, allowing people to "attend" meetings from their homes. Computer bulletin boards open up many new possibilities for homebound individuals (Ferguson 1987; Hazelton 1990). People who live in rural areas can now participate in more meetings per week than are available in the immediate vicinity. Some of these meetings are set up on an ad hoc basis among a small group of callers. Others are scheduled meetings with a more traditional format where callers log in at an appointed time. All of these innovations encourage involvement in 12-step fellowships.

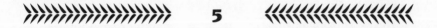

5

The Role of 12-Step Programs in Recovery

- Introduction and Referral to 12-Step Programs
- Newcomers to 12-Step Meetings
- The 90/90 Prescription
- Use of 12-Step Meetings to Promote Recovery
- Interconnection of 12-Step Fellowships

The focus of this book is on facilitating introductions to 12-step programs, either by an individual or by an institution. The terminology preferred by many in the recovering community is *referral* to treatment, in contrast to *introduction* to the Twelve Steps. In the 1989 Narcotics Anonymous membership survey, members were asked how they had been introduced to NA. Forty-seven percent were introduced to the fellowship through hospitals or other institutions; 24% were introduced by a doctor, attorney, judge, member of the clergy, or other professional; and 29% were brought in by another NA member (Narcotics Anonymous 1990). Al-Anon's 1990 survey shows that 42% of all Al-Anon members were introduced by a professional (Al-Anon 1991). (Similar data can be found in Chapter 3 for the most recent AA survey conducted in 1992.)

These findings emphasize the vital importance of social institutions in making referrals to the 12-step programs. (See Section II for further discussion of referral by social institutions.)

Introductions to the 12-step programs can be facilitated in several ways. Ideally, the prospective member should be introduced to an active member of the 12-step community rather than merely receiving a suggestion to attend meetings. A personal introduction to a recovering member of a 12-step group individualizes the referral process and helps the newcomer begin to understand the program. If a personal encounter is not possible as an introduction to the Twelve Steps, an individual can guide someone with a drug or alcohol problem to a meeting. However, to facilitate an appropriate match, the person making the introduction should be familiar with the differences between the fellowships and the various types of meetings. For instance, AA and NA meetings were established for different drug-using populations, although meetings within a community may be more flexible. Al-Anon and Nar-Anon are distinguished by their purpose, which is to help families and friends of alcoholics and other drug users, respectively. Providing the alcoholic-addict or family member with a "Where and When" booklet that lists meeting locations and times and explaining the different types of meetings listed can help the person understand the options and what to expect.

When addicted people first attend a 12-step meeting, it is often through referral from a person or an agency that encourages or even insists on their attendance at meetings. The initial meetings that new members choose are often specific to a facet of their identities. For example, addicted physicians new to the 12-step fellowships tend to seek out meetings with other physicians. Members of a particular racial, ethnic, or age group may initially seek out meetings that closely approximate their own identity. At least initially, people usually feel that they will be more comfortable in meetings with people who are like themselves (Ashery 1979). Soon, however, they realize that their common addiction and the feelings that go with it, along with their spiritual growth, make them all brothers and sisters within the meetings.

The common wisdom of the 12-step programs is that new members should go to 90 meetings in 90 days to get started. The intensive and prolonged immersion in the 12-step fellowships produced by attending meetings daily for 3 months provides the support, reorientation, and beginning behavioral changes that are necessary to break the grip of active addiction and to begin the process of recovery. Without intense and prolonged exposure, the behaviors, feelings, thoughts, and attitudes that provide the foundation for addictive behavior commonly persist, even if they are temporarily obscured under unusual circumstances or with great effort. The intense and prolonged involvement of the 90/90 prescription often initiates profound change in the addicted person. During this time, the alcoholic or addict has the opportunity to meet supportive, abstinent new friends; learn to share thoughts and emotions; begin to understand the steps; learn to have fun without using alcohol or drugs; and begin the quest to find a sponsor. The process of affiliation broadens as people identify with other alcoholics or addicts regardless of background.

Even members of fellowships such as Alcoholics Anonymous with long-term recovery do not know exactly how the 12-step meetings work, and they recognize that many people never allow themselves to "thoroughly follow [the] path." However, members of the 12-step fellowships know from experience and observation that the programs do work for many, regardless of the depth of the problem caused by alcoholism or other addictions. Most members acknowledge that when they first became associated with the 12-step programs, important areas of their lives had become chaotic and unmanageable, including jobs, finances, and relationships with family and friends. Focusing on the immediate problem of addiction often helps solve other related problems. Even when difficult issues need to be addressed, the satisfaction of having one problem under control frequently makes it easier to cope with the others (Alcoholics Anonymous 1989b). A 12-step adage puts it this way: "No problem is so great that alcohol or drugs can't make it worse."

Twelve-step fellowships provide the opportunity to receive help on request, without cost—there are no dues or fees for membership. Whether the initial motivation comes from an individual's desire for recovery or through the intervention of a friend, family member, or professional, access to a 12-step meeting is as close as the nearest telephone. Volunteer members of 12-step programs staff hotline numbers to provide the public with information regarding times and places of meetings. In larger population areas, meetings are held in myriad locations at all hours of the day, from breakfast meetings through midnight fellowships. Rural areas may provide fewer options, but several area meetings generally are spread throughout the week. Whether an individual is seeking help for the first time, a recovering member is facing a crisis and is in fear of relapse, or a family member needs help coping with a loved one's drinking and drug use, a volunteer from a 12-step fellowship is available to provide information and support.

The program of the 12-step fellowships is crucial to the goal of helping alcoholics and addicts on their path to recovery. Many individuals with a history of both alcoholism and drug addiction find AA and NA meetings mutually supportive, because both follow the 12-step program (Nurco et al. 1983). The program is spelled out in the Twelve Steps and strengthened through the policies defined in the Twelve Traditions. The format of the various types of meetings is relatively consistent and predictable from fellowship to fellowship. This consistency makes it possible for alcoholics and addicts to continue on their personal path to recovery regardless of where life leads them. Even though individual meetings often take on a unique personality, the format and issues remain constant for most meetings over long periods of time. The empathy and bonding that is essential in establishing a relationship with a group of people remains with the fellowship rather than with a set of individuals, minimizing the feeling of starting over when attending new meetings.

The peer support that is offered at 12-step meetings is an important aspect of the program. Having a new social system to replace the former drug- or alcohol-involved life-style strongly enhances recovery (Siegel 1988). Addicts who can identify with other members of the fellowship in the quest for recovery offer an acceptance, understanding, and empathy that is not available from the nonaddicted.

The 12-step programs offer an important alternative to what is often termed "white-knuckle sobriety." Although achieving abstinence without external support is certainly possible, maintaining abstinence can be a lonely, painful, and often losing struggle. Typically, 12-step meetings are surprisingly joyful, uplifting gatherings. The emphasis is on "one day at a time" and incremental achievement, with everyone fully realizing the enormous effort required to maintain even small gains. Relapse is recognized as an unfortunate occurrence in the recovery process, rather than as a consummate failure, and the individual who has had the relapse continues to be welcomed with open arms at meetings. Being part of an optimistic recovering fellowship offers an immense advantage over a solitary path toward recovery. The quality of life achieved by supported abstinence strengthens the odds of long-term recovery (Seymour and Smith 1987).

As the process of recovery progresses, some members of 12-step fellowships go to fewer meetings, sometimes just one a week (although this is not recommended). Most long-term members with good sobriety continue to attend two or more meetings each week. In times of stress, or if they feel their abstinence is threatened, members often will step up their meeting attendance.

After individuals become involved in one 12-step fellowship, they may seek out other fellowships. For example, a family member of an alcoholic may start with Al-Anon and then, as the healing process progresses, face up to his or her own addiction to a substance or behavior and attend AA or another appropriate fellowship in addition to Al-Anon. Even more common is the pattern of the alcoholic or addict starting with AA or NA and then attending Al-Anon, Adult Children of Alcoholics, or Co-Dependents Anonymous meetings to confront other issues in their lives; many addicted people grow up and continue to live in families dominated by addiction. However, it is most important to remain active in the primary fellowship of addiction, for which there is no substitute.

As AA's fifth tradition states, "Each group has but one primary purpose—to carry its message to the alcoholic who still suffers." This singleness of purpose has been a vital element in the survival and growth of AA through the years. Other 12-step fellowships have borrowed the steps and traditions of AA and adapted them to their own specific problems. Narcotics Anonymous, in spite of its name, is somewhat more inclusive and welcomes individuals regardless of their drugs of choice. Many other fellowships (including AA) believe that their strength derives in part from the stronger identity and the validity of shared experience that the focus on alcoholism allows. However, in this age of dual addictions, most AA groups welcome to the fellowship people with other addictions, as long as they are or have been active alcoholics and currently have a desire not to drink alcohol.

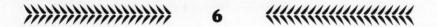
Sponsorship

- Working the Twelfth Step
- Role of the Sponsor
- Finding a Sponsor

The Twelfth Step encourages members to carry the message of recovery to others. Individuals in the fellowships work this step in different ways, including making visits to an addicted person who has asked for help. This outreach activity encourages recovering individuals to redirect their focus to helping others as a way of helping themselves (Chappel 1991). Attending meetings is defined as Twelfth Step work.

Twelfth Step service work by fellowship members is often aimed at referral agencies such as halfway houses, courts, and detoxification and treatment facilities, as well as individual community members. The 12-step fellowships, including AA and NA, are programs of attraction, not proselytization or promotion. AA and NA receive alcoholics and addicts leaving referral institutions and maintain close ties with treatment centers to offer assistance in working with recovering individuals. Fellowship members believe that this outreach is an opportunity to pay back the good that was done for them and to make restitution to the community for any harm they have caused, as outlined in Step Eight (Nurco et al. 1983).

AA's 1992 membership survey underscores the importance of a one-on-one approach—34% of those surveyed were attracted to the group by an AA member. In addition, the larger and more established 12-step groups such as AA, NA, and Al-Anon have organized committees that encourage cooperation with the professional community (Al-Anon 1987; Alcoholics Anonymous 1989a; Narcotics Anonymous 1990). Members of these committees can provide volunteers who will act as temporary sponsors for newcomers.

A larger Twelfth Step commitment to help other addicts is to become a sponsor. AA, NA, and Al-Anon all have pamphlets that discuss the role and responsibilities of sponsorship (Al-Anon 1990; Alcoholics Anonymous 1993; Narcotics Anonymous 1983). Newcomers to 12-step programs benefit from the support and guidance of a sponsor. A sponsor, a 12-step member in stable recovery, develops a personal relationship with a newer member and guides that individual in working the Twelve Steps. In the words of John Chappel (1991), quoting a common AA description, a sponsor is "someone who sees through you and still sees you through."

The sponsorship role is unwritten and informal. An AA pamphlet, "Questions and Answers on Sponsorship" (Alcoholics Anonymous 1993a), provides general suggestions and guidelines for developing sponsor relationships. These suggestions include the sponsor having maintained abstinence for at least 1 year and being the same sex as the person sponsored. Beyond those guidelines, the decision to connect with a particular sponsor is a personal one, with the main goal of the sponsor being to help the newcomer "work the program," to stay sober "one day at a time" and grow in sobriety through the fellowship and the Twelve Steps. NA, being a younger organization, tends to have sponsors with shorter lengths of abstinence, giving rise to more mutual support but potentially greater risk. An NA sponsor also may work with several individuals, building a pyramid of support within the group (Nurco et al. 1983).

Sponsorship is a crucial component of the introductory process. The sponsor provides the pivotal link between an alcoholic-addict or family member and the individual or institution making the referral. Whether an individual is self-referred or enters from a detox-treatment program, learning about the process of recovery and how best to access the 12-step resources is important. Sponsors provide both immediate emergency support and long-term guidance in working the Twelve Steps. (Promoting sponsorship within institutions is an important issue that will be discussed further in Section II.)

A referring institution can help connect new members of 12-step groups to temporary sponsors until the newcomers are familiar enough to find their own sponsors. During many years of membership in a 12-step fellowship, an individual may have one or several sponsors, although usually no more than one at a time. Working the program virtually requires that each member have a sponsor at all times. Not having a sponsor is usually a sign of inadequate (often ambivalent) participation in a 12-step fellowship.

Helping other alcoholics and addicts become abstinent and stay clean and sober is not an act of altruism but is a vital part of a personal program of recovery. This discovery, initially made by Bill Wilson, AA's cofounder, is one of the many unique features of the 12-step process of recovery. Sponsorship is one of the ways this process is expressed in these programs.

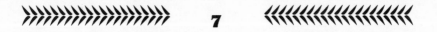

7

Controversies Within the 12-Step Movement

- Autonomy of 12-Step Meetings and Fellowships
- Addiction to More Than One Substance
- Pros and Cons of Compulsory Attendance
- Medication and Its Role in Addiction Treatment
- Substance Abuse and Other Mental Illness
- Spirituality and the 12-Step Programs

As with most human endeavors, the 12-step fellowships are not without controversy. Differences of opinion exist between members attending meetings, between institutional and individual needs, between meetings within a fellowship, and between the different 12-step organizations. Some of the controversies are divisive, and others encourage a healthy exchange of ideas. It is important for individuals and institutions that make referrals to 12-step programs to understand the issues. The following section outlines some of the prominent controversies and discusses the issues involved.

Differences Within the Fellowships and Individual Groups

The 12-step fellowships are highly democratic organizations with few rules. When any issue arises within a 12-step group resulting in a significant dispute among the members, a "group conscience" meeting is called, and the issues are fully discussed. When warranted, volunteers representing both sides of the issue are asked to study the matter and report their findings and thoughts at the next scheduled meeting. A vote of each of the members is taken, and the matter is usually amicably settled, with compromise where indicated. If the matter seems grave enough to the dissenters (such as the issue of holding nonsmoking meetings), they are free to go to other meetings or to start a new one on their own. All that is required to start an AA meeting is "two or more willing alcoholics, a coffee pot, and a place to meet." Other 12-step fellowships are similarly easy to start. The greatest single issue in dispute during recent years seems to have been that of tobacco smoking at meetings. As a result, there are now thousands of nonsmoking 12-step meetings held nationwide and abroad.

Although 12-step fellowships may be specific in their statements about what they do and do not believe and what they do and do not condone, in practice there is considerable latitude within various meetings within individual fellowships. In various geographical regions, individual meetings or local groups within a fellowship may have different rules, definitions, and attitudes. For example, most AA groups will accept members with an addiction to any other abused substance, as long as these individuals are alcoholics also. These AA groups are perfectly comfortable with speakers mentioning their other-than-alcohol drug experiences; other AA meetings do not tolerate mention of any drug other than alcohol. Narcotics Anonymous (NA), on the other hand, welcomes to membership all individuals addicted to any drug (including alcohol).

Attitudes also differ greatly on the question of prescribed medications, with some individual members strictly opposing any use of "mood-altering drugs" and others encouraging appropriate medical treatments by qualified physicians. Both groups oppose nonmedical drug use, including nonmedical use of prescribed controlled substances. However, the fellowship of AA itself takes no official position on these issues or any other, including politics or religion. The only requirement for membership, as stated in the AA Preamble (see Chapter 1) is "a desire to stop drinking," which does not deny but instead encourages members with dual addiction.

Dual Addiction

Dual addiction is the condition of being addicted to more than one substance at the same time—for example, alcoholics who are also addicted to cocaine. To make an appropriate and effective referral, it is important to understand dual addiction and the role it plays in the different 12-step fellowships.

A "pure" alcoholic, or a person limited to an addiction to any one drug, is somewhat unusual today, especially for people under 40. Although polydrug use has become increasingly common and a growing percentage of the recovering community realizes that addiction is addiction regardless of the drug used, dual addiction does present problems within certain fellowships.

In the early 1950s, NA branched off from AA. Some members found that those who were addicted primarily to drugs other than alcohol needed their own program to focus on the disease of addiction without limiting their focus to alcohol. At that time, heroin was the most common nonalcohol drug problem, which helps explain why this fellowship adopted the name "narcotic" rather than the more general term "drug" in its name. Since then, NA has experienced tremendous growth, especially in metropolitan areas on the East and West Coasts, and the focus of NA has broadened to include cocaine, marijuana, and all other drugs. In recent years, a variety of 12-step programs, including Cocaine Anonymous and Marijuana Anonymous, have developed around specific drugs (White and Madara 1992). All of these programs have grown on the basis of demand. AA is by far the largest fellowship, and NA is the largest "drug" fellowship. The other more specific drug-related 12-step groups remain small by comparison. For most addicted individuals, the practical choices are AA or NA or both.

In many ways, this ever-changing diversity is useful. Some people in recovery need to identify with their peers within a framework of drug specificity, such as that provided by Cocaine Anonymous. Addicts spend considerable time thinking about how different they are from other people. The presence of role models, especially others who are further along in recovery from use of the same drug, can be beneficial. The ability to identify with specific role models and to recognize that a specific drug problem exists and can be addressed can be a decisive factor in bringing these addicted individuals into recovery and helping them stay with the program.

A professional medical association, the American Society of Addiction Medicine (ASAM), is composed of physicians with a special interest and expertise in treating addiction. ASAM provides certification for physicians completing a rigorous examination in addiction medicine. (The Appendix includes ASAM's address and telephone number; this organization can provide the names and telephone numbers of member physicians in the United States and internationally.)

Compulsory Attendance

Should attendance at AA meetings be mandated by the courts following conviction of driving while impaired (DWI) or as a condition of probation or parole? Although the issue of compulsory referrals has been argued, several reasons have been presented to support mandated attendance at 12-step meetings. If one assumes that drunk driving is symptomatic of addictive disease, exposure to AA can lead a person toward recovery. A common AA adage is, "Bring the body, the mind will follow."

Referral to 12-step programs from clinical and social model chemical dependency programs is becoming more common. In many cases, attendance at 12-step meetings is incorporated into the inpatient treatment and is a required or recommended element of outpatient treatment. In addiction treatment programs where meeting attendance is a required component of outpatient care, counselors may follow up on meeting attendance by giving clients a special form to be filled in with the date and location of the meeting and signed by the meeting secretary. Courts, probation counselors, and DWI programs often employ similar documentation to verify meeting attendance. There has been some objection, in several locations, that signing the slips implies an affiliation between the 12-step fellowship and the mandating agency. (This controversy and a possible solution to the problem are discussed further in Chapter 11.)

A related objection within the recovering community is that compulsory documentation of meeting attendance runs counter to the AA Eleventh Tradition of anonymity. NA has found that mandated participation appears to be less successful than voluntary participation; the primary benefit of attending 12-step meetings is considered by many to be the individual's desire for help (Nurco et al. 1983). Some 12-step groups have taken a firm position and refuse to sign attendance slips.

A related issue is that smaller, more intimate groups may be inundated with court referrals who do not want to be there and who disrupt the atmosphere of recovery necessary to attract those truly seeking help. For the most part, however, the compulsory referral system has been increasingly accepted and is considered a significant part of 12-step work.

Substitution and Antagonist Therapies

A major focus of this book is to encourage alcohol and drug abuse prevention and treatment programs and other health care organizations—key social institutions—to facilitate high-quality referrals by forming strong links to 12-step programs. One barrier to this introductory process is the resistance of some 12-step groups to accept chemically dependent people who use mind-affecting medicines as part of their treatment. The problem is particularly troublesome when the chemically dependent person being referred is a heroin addict taking methadone or a patient with an anxiety disorder using a benzodiazepine such as Xanax or Valium. Often 12-step members committed to abstinence regard chemical facilitation of recovery through use of Antabuse or naltrexone (antagonists of alcohol and opioids, respectively) as an inappropriate, unreliable aid to progressive lifetime recovery.

Alcoholics in the early stages of recovery or in certain treatment programs may be given Antabuse to prevent early relapse. Antabuse blocks the metabolization of alcohol in the liver. As a result, acetaldehyde accumulates in the body, making alcoholics seriously ill if they drink alcohol. A single dose of Antabuse may produce effects for 5 to 7 days. Although Antabuse can provide protection against impulse drinking, Milam and Ketcham (1981) point out the principal objection to its use within the recovering community:

> The use of Antabuse can distract the alcoholic from assuming responsibility for staying sober. The alcoholic is depending on a drug to keep him [sic] sober, and once the other drug is removed, he will very likely start drinking again. (p. 165)

In a study of alcoholic inpatients' experiences with Antabuse, patients reported little negative reaction in 12-step meetings toward its use. A few participants mentioned that individual members of AA objected to their use of drug therapy, but their decision to continue using it or to continue attending meetings was not affected (Liskow et al. 1990a, 1990b).

Naltrexone works by blocking the receptor sites in the brain that are used by the molecules of opiate and opioid drugs to produce their effects. This narcotic antagonist is taken orally and blocks these receptor sites up to 72 hours after the medicine is taken. During that time, any use of narcotics has no psychoactive effect. Neither Antabuse nor naltrexone is a "psychoactive" drug in the sense that alcohol and heroin are. Neither of these substances produces addiction or euphoria. Instead, they block or discourage the effects of alcohol and narcotic drugs.

Methadone in the treatment of heroin addicts has been a particularly difficult problem for 12-step fellowships precisely because methadone is a psychoactive narcotic. The objections to its use are similar to those voiced about Antabuse and naltrexone, but the opposition within the 12-step community is voiced with greater intensity. Those who have supported methadone treatment and who encourage methadone-treated heroin addicts to use NA and other 12-step fellowships in their recovery emphasize that, as used in treatment, methadone is a medicine, not a "drug." It does not produce euphoria or intoxication, but it does reduce craving and prevent withdrawal symptoms. A regular once-a-day dose of methadone blocks the euphoria of injected heroin or other opiates. In this view, the methadone-maintained patient who refrains from the use of alcohol and other addicting drugs has a clean and sober mind and body, just as does the person who appropriately uses any other medicine. Twelve-step fellowships vary in their receptivity to attendees' disclosures of methadone maintenance therapy (Zweben 1991).

Although there are important differences of opinion on the role of psychoactive medicines in the treatment of addiction, these differences should not obscure important areas of general agreement. Many of the apparent mental illnesses addicted people have when they are actively using alcohol and other drugs diminish and even disappear when they are in recovery and no longer using alcohol and other nonmedical drugs. For this reason, virtually all experts in the field of addiction agree that it is better to first treat addiction and concomitant mental illness without medicines. If the addicted patient can achieve and maintain abstinence and good mental health without using psychoactive medicines, this is by far the most desirable course of action.

Dual Diagnosis

Dual diagnosis, in contrast to dual addiction, refers to substance abusers who, after detoxification, have clinically significant psychopathology independent of their addictive disease. The medical profession now recognizes that 29% of mentally ill people also have substance use disorders, 45% of alcoholics also have a mental disorder or other substance use disorder, and 72% of drug-dependent individuals also have either alcohol use disorder or a mental disorder or both. Dual diagnosis is not unusual; it is at the heart of the treatment of large percentages of those with any of these three groups of illnesses (DuPont 1990a, 1990b; Regier et al. 1990).

Appropriate administration of medicines to manage a psychiatric illness may be indicated for these patients, but the coexistence of chemical dependence needs to be kept in the forefront of their care. If serious and disturbing symptoms of mental illness persist despite nonpharmacological efforts, including regular attendance at 12-step meetings, and if a good response to the use of medical treatments is achieved that does not threaten the patient's recovery, this course of action is often justified. It is generally agreed that the use of psychiatric medicines for dual-diagnosis patients should be considered temporary, with the eventual goal being stability and recovery without their use if that goal can be achieved without worsening the patient's mental disorder.

Some mental illnesses are biological and lifelong, and for these patients, medicines may be needed for a lifetime. Examples include bipolar disorder (manic-depressive disorder) and schizophrenia. A group of physicians in AA has published a pamphlet entitled "The AA Member—Medications and Other Drugs" (Alcoholics Anonymous 1992a) that discusses prescription medication and offers guidelines to help prevent use of medication from becoming a threat to recovery.

The status of anxiety disorders, including panic disorder and generalized anxiety disorder, remains controversial with respect to long-term medicine use. But treatment with medicines that are not controlled substances (such as imipramine and Prozac) are less controversial than the use of benzodiazepines such as Valium and Xanax for people with both an anxiety disorder and alcoholism or drug addiction.

Abuse Potential of Prescribed Medications

Medicines with abuse potential used to treat various illnesses are scheduled under the Controlled Substances Act. These controlled substances include depressants, barbiturates, and benzodiazepines (often used to treat daytime anxiety and nighttime insomnia), stimulants (e.g., amphetamines, no longer widely used in medicine), and narcotics such as codeine and Percodan (used to treat pain).

Among the controlled substances, a substantial difference in abuse potential exists among the drugs. Schedule I drugs have high abuse potential and no approved therapeutic uses. Heroin and LSD are included in this schedule. Schedule II substances have high abuse potential but approved medical uses; cocaine, morphine, and most of the barbiturates and stimulants are in this category. Drugs in Schedule III include Tylenol with codeine. Schedule IV drugs have the lowest level of abuse potential. This group includes the benzodiazepines such as Xanax and Valium. Drug addicts in double-blind research studies generally prefer the drugs in Schedules I and II to those in Schedule IV. However, evidence indicates a substantial abuse potential for benzodiazepines among alcoholics and people addicted to other nonmedical drugs. This same hierarchy of preference is reflected in the price of diverted prescribed medicines on the illicit drug market, with Schedule II drugs commanding far higher prices than Schedule IV drugs.

Most professionals in the addictions field agree that controlled substances should not be used to treat active alcoholics and addicts on an outpatient basis. Whether they should be used to treat alcoholics and addicted individuals with stable recoveries remains controversial among experienced professionals. For example, there is controversy surrounding the use of narcotic analgesics and benzodiazepines in the treatment of anxiety in recovering addicts. It is usually possible to find medicines or nonmedical treatments for these conditions that recovering addicts can use to avoid this controversy.

A report from a group of AA physicians addressing medications recognizes the fact that misuse of certain prescription drugs can threaten sobriety for recovering alcoholics while acknowledging that some people need to use these medications for serious medical problems. Their suggestions for coming to terms with this problem include engendering complete honesty with the prescribing physician about the patient's alcoholism, being totally open with the sponsor, avoiding easy solutions to discomfort, and maintaining active participation in AA. Consulting a physician who specializes in substance abuse problems, especially dual diagnosis with other mental health issues, is highly recommended for addicts who may need to use mind-affecting medicines in their recovery (Alcoholics Anonymous 1992a).

Five key distinctions exist between medical and nonmedical use of potentially abused substances: intent, effect, control, legality, and pattern (DuPont 1990b, 1990c). Medical treatment is associated with a serious, diagnosed illness. Legitimate medical treatment results in improvement in the user's life, is legal, is controlled not only by the user but also by the fully informed physician, and is used in a stable and responsible pattern. Nonmedical substance use is the opposite. It is for pleasure or "self-treatment," it makes the user's life worse, it is illegal (except for alcohol use by adults), it is exclusively controlled by the user (subject to access), and it is typically used in chaotic and irresponsible patterns. In a word, alcohol and other drugs are used "addictively," whereas medicines are used "medically." Medical professionals who treat addicted people, fellowship members, and sponsors who work with medically treated addicted people should all be aware of these distinctions between medical and nonmedical substance use. If these guidelines are followed, there is seldom a conflict between the use of medicines and participation in 12-step fellowships, providing that those people who are in treatment are honest with their physicians and their 12-step sponsors.

The controversies surrounding the use of controlled substances by recovering addicts, and the use of medicines to treat addiction itself, must be kept separate from two conclusions with wide acceptance in both the addiction treatment field and the recovering community:

1. Controlled substances generally should not be prescribed in the treatment of active addicts in outpatient settings because of the high risk that the controlled substances will contribute to the addiction problem.
2. Noncontrolled medicines used to treat physical illness (including pain control) and mental illness (other than addiction itself), such as depression, anxiety disorders, and psychotic disorders, generally are not a problem for addicted people. The medicines are often vital to recovery itself, because people with inadequately treated illnesses often do poorly in their recovery programs if their illnesses remain untreated. This position has been officially endorsed by AA (Alcoholics Anonymous 1992a). All physicians and pharmacists know which medicines are controlled substances and which are not.

In contrast to these areas of general agreement among physicians and members of the 12-step fellowships, two areas of disagreement remain. The first is the use of controlled substances in the outpatient treatment of any recovering person, even one who has a stable abstinence from the nonmedical use of alcohol and other drugs. The second is the use of any medicine, including medicines not covered under the Controlled Substances Act (such as Antabuse, naltrexone, and antidepressants) to treat addiction itself or to prevent relapses. Although these important areas remain unsettled, the existence of these disagreements should not detract from the far greater areas where broad agreement has been reached.

Medication Issues in
12-Step Referral

To provide an educated introduction to appropriate 12-step meetings, referral agencies and individuals need to be aware of these conflict-generating medical issues. Matching an individual with a knowledgeable sponsor is often crucial when special needs arise in controversial areas of 12-step programs.

As was discussed in the previous section, the use of psychoactive drugs can be controversial in 12-step programs. The official AA position in conference-approved literature is that members should take prescribed medicine if needed (Alcoholics Anonymous 1992a). However, some 12-step meeting groups do not consider members "clean and sober" when they are using any psychoactive medication. Cases of adverse treatment consequences, even suicide, have resulted from well-meaning 12-step members dissuading individuals from taking prescribed medications.

From a clinical perspective, the legitimate medicating of an independent psychiatric disorder with a noncontrolled substance is no more a violation of a chemical-free philosophy than prescribing penicillin for an infection or insulin for diabetes. However, some individuals within the recovering community consider the prescription and use of psychoactive medication as a violation of the 12-step precepts. This lack of tolerance can place an individual who needs the support of 12-step interaction *and* psychiatric medication in an untenable position. To continue effective psychiatric treatment, some individuals feel constrained not to mention their medication in meetings or to their sponsors. This lack of honesty can be detrimental to recovery. When referring a dually diagnosed patient or client, it is important for a clinician to find a 12-step group that is tolerant of legitimate medication needs and to continue to educate the 12-step fellowship on the nature and treatment of dual diagnosis. Interactive support of the patient's understanding of the need for medication can counteract the effects of well-meaning but intolerant individuals within the group who may try to talk the patient out of taking necessary medicine.

Total honesty is the best preventive measure. This means that the patient, the physician, the sponsor, and the patient's family all need to know the whole truth about the patient's chemical dependence and all use of psychoactive medicines. The alcoholic's or addict's dishonesty toward any of these people is a serious adverse sign for which all participants need to be vigilant. It is no accident that many AA members are skeptical of physicians who say, "Trust me, I'm a doctor." When it comes to psychoactive medicine use by chemically dependent individuals, such "trust" often has been part of the addiction, not part of the recovery. To guard against such a possibility, openness and honesty for everyone involved is essential.

Spirituality and Religion

From AA's very beginning when it emerged from the Oxford Group movement, the spiritual focus of the 12-step fellowships has caused controversy. AA's contemporary spirituality is often confused with the practice of organized religion. Bill W., cofounder of Alcoholics Anonymous, was originally skeptical of his friend Ebbie T., a former heavy drinker who based his newly found sobriety on "getting religion." Once he himself stopped drinking and became acquainted with members of the Oxford Group, however, Bill W. recognized similarities between early Christianity and what was to become AA philosophy. One alcoholic talking to another constituted a meeting, a one-on-one "conversion" of alcoholics. The Oxford Group, although nondenominational, was based on the theology of first-century Christianity. Passages from the New Testament book of James inspired the emphasis on "good works" that drove Bill W. and Dr. Bob to seek out alcoholics and even offer them lodging during their treatment. They also learned that the "good works" were for themselves, in that working with other alcoholics was the best (and perhaps only) way of maintaining their sobriety "one day at a time." Because of the early AA association with the Oxford Group, initially the Catholic Church identified the AA movement as Protestant and forbade its members from any association with the organization. Eventually a Catholic priest investigated an early AA meeting and gave the recovery process a clean bill of health from the church's point of view. AA lost much of its religious focus in the first few years but retains a profoundly spiritual message (Kurtz 1987; Robertson 1988). The acceptance of this nonreligious but spiritual philosophy is evident in the establishment of 12-step meetings in diverse social and cultural areas, both in the United States and throughout the world.

From the beginning, some pioneers in the AA movement strongly opposed even the slightest theological dimension of the Twelve Steps. This opposition is well documented in Dr. Earle M.'s *Physician, Heal Thyself! 35 Years of Adventures in Sobriety by an AA "Old-Timer"* (1989). Earle M., a physician, had difficulty with the religious overtones of AA, especially the wording of several of the Twelve Steps, although he felt that "despite my criticisms of [these steps] I believed that they were valuable" (p. 86). A final revision of the Twelve Steps that deinstitutionalized the concept of God took place before the "Big Book" went to press. The phrase "Power greater than ourselves" was substituted for God in Step Two, and "God *as we understood Him*" in Steps Three and Eleven.

Twelve-step programs do not adhere to a single concept of a deity but rather to a Higher Power that can be defined by the individual member, perhaps with the aid of the sponsor and fellow members. For those with a traditional religious background, that power may be a traditional one; for others, the Higher Power can take on more personal characteristics. Some individuals, especially as newcomers, are content with believing that the 12-step group itself is the power greater than themselves. "They were staying sober when I couldn't" is a frequent comment by newcomers. Traditional 12-step meetings attempt to keep references to specific religious beliefs to a minimum, emphasizing that although spiritual experiences and values are essential, discussion of personal religious views is inappropriate at 12-step meetings.

Although AA split from the earlier Oxford Group, today AA is worldwide, and the Oxford Group has all but disappeared. Alternative groups that have diverged radically from AA since its founding in the 1930s have, despite their temporary notoriety, remained small and mostly disappeared after a few years. NA, Al-Anon, and Adult Children of Alcoholics are prominent exceptions to this generalization. The durability of AA is eloquent testimony to the breadth and depth of the needs AA meets for millions of people. This reality reflects the strength of the program and should give pause to outside observers who seek, however benevolently, to improve on the AA program.

The mention of God "as we understood Him" or a Higher Power in the Twelve Steps, and the common practice of reciting the Lord's Prayer to close meetings, can make acceptance difficult for members of non-Christian faiths or those who reject organized religion. Among Orthodox Jews, entering a Gentile house of worship is prohibited, making attendance in church halls problematic. The Jewish Alcoholics, Chemically Dependent Persons and Significant Others (JACS) Foundation described in Chapter 13 is an example of an organization that helps overcome some of these barriers.

Atheist and agnostic meetings have been formed in response to concerns about religious connotations perceived in the 12-step programs. Secular Organizations for Sobriety (SOS) and Methods of Moderation (MOM) are examples of alternative recovery groups, based on the Twelve Steps and open to individuals of any belief system. Another alternative, not based on the traditional Twelve Steps, is Rational Recovery (RR), a cognitive-behavioral self-help program based on the principles of rational-emotive therapy developed by Albert Ellis. RR emphasizes self-reliance, rational thought, and altered behavior during events that trigger drinking (Hall 1990).

Identity groups other than atheists may be deterred by the perceived religious connotation of AA. This common criticism is confounded because AA, and other 12-step programs, are spiritually based but not religiously oriented. Gay men and lesbians often hesitate to participate in an organization that can be perceived as holding the same Christian values that may censure their life-style. Increasingly, AA and other 12-step meetings started by members who are gay men or lesbians are identified as such in area directories.

The State of Maryland recently was embroiled in a court case addressing the issue of mandatory referral to AA programs following a DWI conviction. As reported in the *Baltimore City Paper* (Lamb-Korn 1991), the American Civil Liberties Union (ACLU) and RR systems testified on behalf of a bill to offer alternatives to treatment programs that use "religious or spiritual elements as an integral aspect" (p. A1). The ACLU argued that AA meets the legal definition of a religion. On the opposing side, Maryland state officials argued that AA's spiritual orientation is not the same as a secular religion and therefore does not affect an individual's civil liberties (Lamb-Korn 1991). Maryland currently mandates referral to a self-help program, allowing individuals to choose groups that best meet their needs.

Twelve-step beliefs do not actually conform to the definition of an established religion in that they are not a codified belief system. Instead, the 12-step fellowships teach the vital role of spirituality, an acknowledgment of a force outside of the individual (Chappel 1990). Unlike conflicting religious practices, and furthering Chappel's ideas, a person can be a Presbyterian AA member, a Buddhist NA member, an agnostic Al-Anon member, an atheist adult child of an alcoholic, or any other combination. Finding one's Higher Power or "God as [we] understood Him" for religious and nonreligious members alike is essential for growth in the 12-step program. Addressing the role that spirituality takes in the recovery process is an important part of introducing someone to 12-step fellowships. (AA recognizes this in Chapter 4 of the "Big Book" (1976), "We Agnostics.") Agencies and individuals making referrals need to understand these issues to avoid this common stumbling block to understanding 12-step programs.

Resolution of these conflicts is not needed, nor is it possible; rather, they need to be clearly recognized and directly acknowledged. If we use the bridge metaphor for the introduction to 12-step programs, the controversies may be considered checkpoints along the way for some individuals, but they need not be barriers to crossing. Agencies and individuals introducing alcoholics and addicts to 12-step fellowships must understand these potential obstacles to guide newcomers to the other side of the bridge, the side where recovery lies.

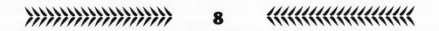 **8**

Building Bridges to 12-Step Fellowships

- Ten Steps to Building the Bridge
- Bridge-Building Checklist

Alcoholics and addicts—together with their families, friends, and acquaintances—have difficulty identifying addiction as a serious, lifelong disease with biopsychosocial roots. Denial is the primary obstacle. Often denial is so strong and pervasive that even concerned professionals fail to identify a person bound by addiction or a family member tragically affected by a relative's substance abuse. Identification and acknowledgment of addiction are the first and most difficult steps on the road to recovery. This chapter focuses on the next step in the process, one that also can prove challenging: once the addiction has been recognized and acknowledged, how can an individual find and use a 12-step program as part of the recovery process?

Virtually everyone in America today has heard of Alcoholics Anonymous. But most people do not understand what AA is, how it works, or how to find out more about the program. Even fewer people know of the array of 12-step programs that are available today. For example, some experts in the field of addiction do not realize that Alateen, a part of Al-Anon, is a fellowship of teenagers affected by someone else's alcoholism and not a group for adolescents seeking help for their own problems with alcohol. The fundamental distinction between organized, professional treatment of addiction on the one hand and 12-step fellowships on the other is seldom made in most people's thinking about addiction.

To take full advantage of the enormous capability of the 12-step programs, every individual who routinely comes in contact with alcoholism and addiction should learn to recognize the disease and know how to make an appropriate referral to a 12-step program. Especially in major social institutions, organized efforts are needed to teach members how to identify addiction and to make effective referrals to 12-step fellowships.

The following 10-point list outlines recommendations for social institutions to strengthen the introductory process.

1. A common way to encourage an introduction to a 12-step meeting is by giving an individual the telephone number of a fellowship and providing access to a telephone. It is important that the individual seeking help make the call rather than a friend, family member, or professional. Calling one of these numbers connects the caller with a volunteer who has information about where and when meetings are held locally. This technique is appropriately used by family members as well as institutions. Meeting lists are available through each of the 12-step programs.

2. Social institutions need to educate clients about addiction and recovery directly through 12-step literature, lectures, discussion groups, referral counselors, and media materials. An abundance of high-quality information is available through printed materials, audiotapes, and videotapes. The fellowships themselves provide explanatory literature at nominal cost. In addition to direct messages about the 12-step philosophy of recovery, institutions can incorporate indirect background information about the programs. Using common AA phrases

such as "One Day at a Time" and "First Things First" in the counseling process or posting the Serenity Prayer in an entryway introduces important 12-step concepts and familiarizes newcomers with the language commonly used in fellowship meetings.

3. Everyone who represents one of the major social institutions described in Section II needs to be personally familiar with 12-step meetings. For example, teachers and physicians need to attend four or five (or more) open 12-step meetings to become familiar with the basic agenda and format. They also need to familiarize themselves with the philosophy of the 12-step movement through the available literature. Professional education should include information on alcoholism and addiction prevention and treatment, including training about the 12-step groups. In many 12-step fellowships, professionals are welcomed at open meetings as "friends" of the alcoholic or addict.

4. Social institutions are encouraged to hold educational meetings about the 12-step fellowships. For example, some employee assistance programs (EAPs) offer educational meetings for employees and families in which representatives of the 12-step fellowships describe program and meeting formats. Institutions can incorporate information about the 12-step groups in their ongoing education, training, and conferences for the public, patients, and staff.

5. If appropriate, on-site meetings should be built into the inherent structure of the institution. These meetings, referred to as H and I (hospital and institutional) or treatment facility meetings, are not true community meetings open to everyone. Instead, these meetings build a bridge between the institution and 12-step meetings in the community at large. H and I meetings are held in many inpatient drug and alcohol treatment programs and in correctional facilities. These meetings effectively introduce individuals to the 12-step philosophy of recovery.

6. Social institutions should encourage regular in-house 12-step meetings. Holding meetings on the premises facilitates access

and demonstrates institutional support for the 12-step programs. It is important to allow 12-step fellowships to hold their
own meetings to preserve independence and nonaffiliation
with the institution. Schools, churches, worksites, correctional
facilities, and other institutions can provide space for regular
meetings.

7. An excellent referral strategy for institutions is to identify staff
    members to serve in a liaison capacity between the institution
    and the 12-step communities. If they are 12-step members, care
    needs to be taken to keep the two roles separate. Both 12-step
    fellowship members and others are useful in this facilitative
    role to avoid its being relegated to fellowship members alone.
    EAPs in the workplace and SAPs (student assistance programs)
    in schools provide useful introductory services. Supervisors
    and teachers suggest use of the EAP or SAP, and the counselor
    in turn introduces employees or students and their families to
    appropriate 12-step groups.

8. An effective introduction often can be made by connecting the
    individual with an active fellowship member. EAPs frequently
    match an employee with an "old-timer" from a 12-step pro-
    gram who works in the same company. Members with longtime
    knowledge of the 12-step fellowships can answer questions and
    accompany newcomers to their first meetings. When selecting
    a meeting, it is important to consider the background and
    identity of a newcomer. Special meetings for beginners,
    women, young people, or gay men and lesbians should be con-
    sidered for initial meetings to help the newcomer feel a con-
    nection to the group.

9. Social institutions increasingly are requiring addicted people
    to attend 12-step programs as a consequence of positive drug
    or alcohol tests or admission of drug and/or alcohol use. The
    DWI programs of many states use this mandatory referral pro-
    cess, requiring participants to show evidence of attendance by
    obtaining a signed slip at each meeting. EAP counselors are
    beginning to use required 12-step attendance as a method to
    involve alcoholics and addicts in the fellowships. As we men-

tioned earlier, some 12-step meetings are balking at required attendance and refusing to sign attendance slips. To avoid an unfortunate situation, organizations should check in advance to determine whether a meeting will welcome individuals who are required to attend.

10. Referral goes beyond sending a person to a meeting. Introducing someone to 12-step fellowships also means responding to concerns that are raised following meeting attendance. Answering questions and providing support and feedback to a novice is important. If the initial meeting does not meet the needs of the newcomer, the person making the referral needs to discuss the problem and be prepared to ask an experienced fellowship member to help out and perhaps to find a more appropriate group. Only by forming a solid link with the 12-step community will an introduction be likely to take hold and thrive.

Each social institution needs to review its current practices periodically and implement as many of these 10 recommendations as appropriate (Table 2).

Table 2.   A checklist—introduction techniques to 12-step programs for social institutions

_____   1. Provide information describing 12-step fellowships and encourage initial phone contact with 12-step groups.

_____   2. Hold educational meetings on the 12-step fellowships for staff members and others associated with the institution.

_____   3. Encourage staff to become familiar with 12-step programs by attending meetings, both in-house and in the community.

_____   4. Hold beginner meetings in the institution.

_____   5. Build 12-step meetings and philosophy into the institutional structure.

_____   6. Hold regular 12-step meetings in-house.

_____   7. Identify key staff to make introductions to meetings.

_____   8. Provide temporary sponsors for new attendees at both in-house and community meetings.

_____   9. Include 12-step meetings in institutional requirements.

_____ 10. Follow up referrals of new attendees to 12-step fellowships.

Section II

Institutions That Encounter Addiction: Problems, Solutions, and Recommendations

Institutions are on one side of the referral bridge, and the 12-step programs are on the other. When an institution introduces addicted people and/or their families to one of the 12-step fellowships, it has helped them cross the bridge to recovery. The major institutions that make these introductions are discussed in the following chapters. These are institutions that meet human needs and confront addictions. They include the institutions of the family, health care, substance abuse treatment, criminal justice, religion, and the workplace.

The checklist of referral techniques found in Chapter 8 can be used by each of these social institutions to assess and to facilitate the process of introduction—of crossing the bridge to recovery. The institutions, and the unique roles they play in the recovery process, are the focus of the following chapters.

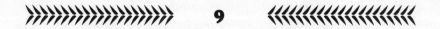 **9**

The Family

- The Family's Role in Addiction and Recovery
- The Problem of Co-Dependence

Most people live in families, and families live in communities. Within the last 20 years in the United States, however, "family" has become increasingly difficult to define. The typical nuclear family consisting of father, mother, and two children has given way to diverse households— single-parent families, childless couples, and more or less stable households consisting of unrelated members. As a conservative estimate, there were more than 93 million households in the United States in 1990. For the purposes of this discussion, a family is defined as a group of individuals living together in a more or less enduring household. By this definition, a family could be three generations under one roof, two sets of children merged through remarriage, a couple living together, or even a relatively stable group home. A community is composed of many such households, most of which are stable and cohesive, living in relative proximity to each other.

Addiction is a disease that affects everyone close to an addict, especially family members. No matter how strong the family or community, alcoholism and addiction make households and

71

neighborhoods chaotic and unmanageable. This state of disorganization is often described as "dysfunctional." Everyday behaviors that worked reasonably well prior to addiction become destructive to the human potential of family members or the community. Families need clear guidelines to recognize substance abuse, and they need practical and available responses to addiction when it is identified. Addiction often grows out of behavior that seems normal and acceptable. For example, alcoholism can develop from "social drinking." Addicted people deny their behaviors and the consequences of those behaviors, making it difficult for families and communities to identify addictive diseases. Addiction, though it can develop in any family or any community, is more likely to occur in families and communities already less able to cope with problems.

Alcoholics and addicts frequently are incapacitated by denial of their problems. Families can be blinded by denial. However, families—especially through a professionally guided intervention—can help the alcoholic or addict break through denial. The first outcome of a structured intervention may be a traditional inpatient addiction treatment program. In some cases, direct referral to and involvement in 12-step fellowships may start the individual and his or her family along the path to lifelong recovery. The 12-step fellowships publish several pamphlets for families with one or more members struggling with a chemical dependency problem. Twelve-step fellowships that focus on friends and family members of the alcoholic or addict, such as Al-Anon, Alateen, and Nar-Anon, can be instrumental in helping those close to the addicted person overcome their own denial. Association with others in similar situations helps family members who have become enablers understand their own roles and ways they effectively can help themselves (Al-Anon 1969).

Families affected by chemical dependence are often dysfunctional and unable to promote the well-being of all family members. Family members unwittingly can impede an alcoholic's or addict's desire to become drug-free. Each member assumes a role enabling the addict to pursue addiction. The family frequently adopts stereotyped counterproductive interactions to cope with the addicted person (Cermak 1990). When the alcoholic or addict enters treatment or becomes invested in a 12-step fellowship, the family members may perceive their unity or self-esteem as threatened. Unless they also get help, the family may become even more dysfunctional when the addict approaches recovery. Family members of addicted people are called "co-dependent," meaning that they share the disease with the addicted family member. Usually the co-dependent family member has become "addicted to the addict," meaning that the family member's life and self-esteem are dependent on the addicted person's behavior (McGovern and DuPont 1992). Co-dependent family members may consciously or unconsciously attempt to return the family system to its more familiar survival structure of imbalance by sabotaging the addict's treatment or recovery (Kaufman 1985). To overcome this common problem, virtually all addiction treatment programs include family members in all stages of the treatment process, referring them to family-based 12-step fellowships.

Even without formalized inclusion of family members in a structured addiction treatment plan, those with close relationships to an addicted or alcoholic member need to work through their co-dependence and become aware of their behavior, which promotes the addict's abuse of alcohol and other drugs. This behavior is called "enabling," because the family members enable the addiction to continue. Typical enabling behavior involves making excuses for the addicted individual at work or among friends. Twelve-step support groups such as Al-Anon and Alateen are specifically organized to offer support to the families and friends of alcoholics. Similar groups, such as Nar-Anon, have been formed to provide the same service for families of addicts. Co-dependents Anonymous is a rapidly growing fellowship for people who are "addicted to an addict."

AA reports that one member in five is introduced to the 12-step programs by a family member (Alcoholics Anonymous 1993a). Those close to an alcoholic or addict have a unique opportunity to affect the recovery of a loved one through introduction to the Twelve Steps.

Health Care Systems and Substance Abuse Treatment Facilities

- The Role of Health Care Providers
- The Role of Alcohol and Drug Abuse Treatment
- Twelve-Step Meetings in the Community
- Hospital and Institutional Meetings
- Transitional Living Programs

Health care professionals and institutions are instrumental in identifying and treating substance abuse disorders. In 1990, health care costs in the United States totaled $666.2 billion, or 12.2% of the gross national product (GNP) (Levit et al. 1991). By the year 2000, health care costs are projected to rise to $1.6 trillion, or 16.4% of GNP (Sonnefeld et al. 1991). In 1988, the economic cost of alcohol abuse was estimated at $85.8 billion and the cost of drug abuse at $58.3 billion (Rice et al. 1990). The cost of direct and support costs for alcoholism treatment equaled 10% of the total cost of alcohol abuse in 1985. This cost included $2.3 billion for patients whose primary diagnosis was alcohol abuse, and $700 million for patients with a secondary diagnosis of alcohol abuse who were hospitalized an average of 2.8 days longer than patients who were not diagnosed as alcohol abusers (Rice and Kelman 1989).

In terms of indirect costs, the morbidity (or value of lost productivity) of those who abuse alcohol was estimated at $27.4 billion in 1985, and the morbidity of those who abuse drugs was estimated at $6 billion. The other component of indirect costs, the mortality costs, is the product of the number of deaths associated with alcohol or drug abuse and the expected value of an individual's future earnings if he or she had not died prematurely. For alcohol abuse, the estimated mortality cost was $24 billion in 1985, and for drug abuse, it was estimated at $2.6 billion. Deaths associated with alcohol abuse represented 1.5 million person-years lost in 1985 (Rice et al. 1991).

Many of the costs of alcoholism and addiction reach beyond the costs of treatment to include other related health consequences such as liver cirrhosis, cancer, motor vehicle crashes, and other trauma. If alcoholism and addiction were identified and treated earlier in the addiction process, related medical costs could be reduced (Gordis 1991).

In an effort to contain these enormous costs, health care workers need to recognize alcohol and other drug abuse and be prepared to make appropriate referrals to professional treatment and 12-step programs. A recent study of health care costs associated with formal alcoholism treatment showed that total health care costs of those receiving treatment declined by 23% to 55% after 6 months compared with their highest pretreatment levels. In addition, alcoholics who received treatment incurred medical costs that were 24% less than those of untreated alcoholics over a 4-year period (Holder and Blose 1992). Primary care physicians, nurses, social workers, therapists, and all other health care workers involved in direct patient contact should be educated in methods to identify and confront substance abuse. Although the process itself is accomplished on an individual basis, the health organization (whether it is a hospital, emergency room, private medical or mental health practice, health maintenance organization [HMO], or publicly funded clinic) needs to recognize and support efforts to confront the problems of alcoholism and addiction.

Physicians are an important link in the introductory process. They are frequently in a unique position to offer guidance to patients seeking treatment for an illness related or unrelated to drinking or drug use. Specific screening instruments are available that provide objectivity to the assessment process (U.S. Department of Health and Human Services 1990c). Individuals in recovery are often disappointed that their physicians did not recognize their disease or know how to help them overcome it. The Betty Ford Center, an alcohol and drug addiction treatment facility, discovered that only 1% of the 19,000 individuals treated in the last 10 years were referred by physicians (Vance 1992). AA or NA members sometimes find that their personal physicians have little knowledge of what takes place at 12-step meetings, about potentially addicting prescription medications, or about recovery. The 1992 AA membership survey revealed that only 7% of members were referred by their physicians (Alcoholics Anonymous 1993b). In such cases, 12-step members increasingly "sponsor their physicians"—that is, they educate their own doctors about their personal recovery through AA or NA and help them understand the importance of the fellowships. From the point of view of many physicians, the 12-step programs do not fit with the scientific basis of traditional medical practice. The spirituality aspects and life-style changes that are central to the 12-step programs, although essential to the recovery process, do not conform to scientific inquiry compatible with a clinician's background (Miller and Ries 1990).

The National Institute on Drug Abuse (NIDA) and the National Institute on Alcohol Abuse and Alcoholism (NIAAA) have funded grants for health professionals in substance abuse research and education (National Institute on Alcohol Abuse and Alcoholism 1991; Williams 1990). Included in some of these training programs is a focus on the role of 12-step programs in recovery.

Health care workers themselves are not immune to the impact of alcoholism and addiction. Many of them have become members of 12-step fellowships and, in addition, have formed recovery groups centered around their professions. Examples of such groups include International Doctors in AA, International Nurses Anonymous, and International Pharmacists Anonymous (White and Madara 1992).

Under the umbrella of health care, alcohol and drug treatment programs provide specialized services for those with the diseases of alcoholism or addiction. According to the National Drug and Alcoholism Treatment Unit Survey 1987 Final Report, 6,866 inpatient treatment facilities served a population of more than 614,000 clients. In addition, 2,526 programs provided treatment on an outpatient basis (National Institute on Drug Abuse 1989b). Drug and alcohol treatment programs can be part of a comprehensive hospital setting, or they can be autonomous institutions. Nearly all recovery programs offer aftercare or continuing care to clients leaving the facility and returning to the community (Office of National Drug Control Policy 1990).

Alcohol and other drug treatment centers are professionally staffed, usually by health professionals including physicians (psychiatrists and other clinicians), psychologists, social workers, nurses, and specially trained addiction counselors. Addiction treatment takes place on either an inpatient or an outpatient basis. Inpatient treatment is usually brief, often lasting 28 days or less. Outpatient treatment can take the form of aftercare following inpatient treatment, or it can be an alternative to inpatient treatment. In the latter case, outpatient addiction treatment often lasts 4 to 10 weeks or longer, often involving 20 or more hours a week of care.

Psychotherapy (both group and individual) can last longer but is usually less intensive, often meeting once a week for an hour or two. Aftercare following inpatient or intensive outpatient addiction treatment may continue up to a year or even longer, although the frequency may decline to an hour or two per week as a person's recovery becomes stronger. Professional addiction treatment can be relatively expensive, whether paid for by the individual, by health insurance, or through public agencies. Nevertheless, compared to active addiction, and to the extent that it is successful, addiction treatment is a bargain compared to the health care and social costs of continuing addiction. Often formal addiction treatment is the vital first step in the process of lifelong recovery.

Many inpatient drug and alcohol treatment programs are based on a treatment program that originated in the 1950s at Willmar State Hospital in Minnesota. That program, based on the Twelve Steps of Alcoholics Anonymous and lasting 28 days, became known as the Minnesota model. It is now the dominant form of private treatment for addiction in the United States (Office of National Drug Control Policy 1990). Private chemical dependence treatment programs share the core characteristics of the original Minnesota model, including the use of a multidisciplinary treatment team, an individualized treatment plan, family involvement in the treatment process, and the 12-step disease concept of addiction and recovery (Hazelden Foundation 1990). The duration of inpatient stay in addiction treatment now varies widely, depending on the needs of the alcoholic or addicted patient and on insurance and/or other funding available. The essential feature of these programs is not that they last "28 days" but that they follow the treatment approach used by Hazelden treatment programs, the Betty Ford Center, and other well-known programs.

Substance abuse treatment is provided by licensed health care professionals (such as physicians, psychologists, social workers, and counselors) who are paid for their work, often through public tax funds or by private health insurance. Addiction treatment programs, many of which now employ professionals who are themselves members of 12-step fellowships, are organized in a way similar to other health care institutions licensed in their communities and run by paid staffs of professionals and administrators.

Treatment programs have both inpatient and outpatient components with specified periods of treatment—for example, 28 days of inpatient addiction treatment, or 10 weeks or more of outpatient treatment. Some addiction treatment programs are for-profit and others are nonprofit organizations; some addiction treatment programs are public agencies and others are private institutions. All are distinctively different from the 12-step fellowships that are not fee-for-service programs, do not have set durations of treatment, and are not licensed by any governmental agency. Most of the organized addiction treatment programs in the United States now use 12-step fellowships in their programs. The Minnesota model of the inpatient residential addiction treatment center has become the prototype of an organized social institution, building into its established programming 12-step meetings for addicted people and their families.

Many addicted people and their relatives are so overcome by shame and turmoil that they are unable initially to use 12-step programs, preferring the authority and security of a professional addiction treatment program. Once they have gotten professional treatment and (through this treatment) been introduced to the 12-step fellowships, they continue to attend meetings in their own communities.

Most inpatient drug treatment centers now use the 12-step programs of AA and NA as an important component of treatment aftercare. The standard alcohol treatment program as outlined in the *New England Journal of Medicine* includes referral to AA following inpatient rehabilitation (Klerman 1989). During the last week of treatment, a patient is matched with a volunteer from the patient's community whose role is to introduce the recovering individual to local AA or NA meetings. At the nationally known Betty Ford Center and Hazelden, for example, the treatment programs are designed around the 12-step philosophy. AA and NA meetings are an integral part of the daily schedule, and the aftercare component of recovery emphasizes participation in 12-step meetings. Modern outpatient alcohol and drug abuse treatment programs usually include attendance at AA, NA, or CA meetings in the ongoing process of recovery.

The Phoenix Adolescent Recovery Center, a private, extended-care service for chemically dependent adolescents, provides another example. This program incorporates AA and NA as integral parts of its recovery program. Starting on day one, residents of this program attend 12-step meetings in the community, attending a minimum of nine meetings per week. They are responsible for recruiting their own sponsors. Although they may attend any community meeting, those targeted toward young people are encouraged. As the residents work through the Phoenix House program, they are required to attend community meetings solo and then speak at and chair community 12-step meetings. The adolescents also participate in social activities sponsored by 12-step fellowships, including dances, retreats, and Alco-thons (a marathon of activities occurring during a particularly vulnerable time, such as New Year's Eve). The goal of the Phoenix adolescent treatment program, facilitated by regular attendance at 12-step meetings, is to make major life changes that enhance recovery (C. Policano, personal communication, February 1991).

Initially, AA meetings were brought into many hospital treatment settings because state institutions could not take patients out into the community. Patients who had experience only with institutional meetings found the transition to fellowships outside the hospital setting difficult. In addition to the stress associated with returning to the drug-using environment, the former patient was expected to depend on a group of strangers for a support system.

Greater efforts are now being made to include patients in regular community fellowships during alcohol and drug treatment. To accomplish this, staff members accompany patients to fellowship meetings that are determined in advance to be the most appropriate. This determination may be based on proximity to the patient's home or workplace, ethnic or income composition of the meeting participants, or other identity factors. Development of a stable support system prior to leaving the addiction treatment center makes the transition to the home environment and abstinence more successful. Few treatment programs, especially those based on the Minnesota model, hold 12-step meetings exclusively on campus. For instance, at Hazelden, the only on-site 12-step meeting is held during the lunch hour for employees. Patients at Hazelden go into the community to 12-step meetings from the beginning of their residential treatment. This approach from the beginning of treatment facilitates the transition to participation after discharge.

In locations where escorting patients to community meetings is not feasible—for example, in drug treatment centers that work with alcoholic or addicted offenders from the criminal justice system—community meetings can be brought into the institution. AA holds two types of meetings in treatment facilities. The first type of meeting is structured to meet the particular needs of patients in drug or alcohol treatment. These meetings are not listed in the local directory and are not open to the community, although members of a local 12-step meeting may be invited to attend as speakers. The second type of meeting is regular AA meetings attended both by AA members and by patients at the facility. In this case, meeting space and coffee are provided by the institution, and local AA members can choose to attend regular meetings at the facility. These meetings are open to the community and are published in the local meeting directory. In-house meetings offer an optimal opportunity for recovering patients to associate with a support system within the treatment experience that will facilitate the transition to the wider community. AA and other 12-step fellowships provide guidelines for both types of meetings (Alcoholics Anonymous 1987). One important issue is the avoidance of accepting financial support from the institution. Groups are encouraged by the fellowship to pay for their coffee and, if appropriate, for use of the meeting space.

Institutions need to prepare patients for participation in 12-step aftercare. Recovering addicts and alcoholics emphasize the need to bring meetings into the institution and not just assume that professionals are communicating about the 12-step programs to patients and clients. Newcomers need to know what to expect at a group meeting. They need to know what meetings are and what they are not. For instance, former patients who have been involved in individual counseling and group psychotherapy need to understand that the discussions at 12-step meetings focus more on the solutions to achieving abstinence and maintaining sobriety through the Twelve Steps and are less involved with specific issues involving relationships and employment concerns.

Important dimensions to meeting interactions include discouragement of cross-talk (a direct response to a person's comments that can result in confrontation), constraints on interpreting comments of other members, minimization of confrontation, verbal reinforcement of contributions to the discussion, and discouragement of one member dominating the meeting.

Hospital and Institutional (H and I) Meetings

H and I meetings provide a formal mechanism for preparing clients to attend 12-step meetings. These meetings are more directed and structured than regular AA meetings. Their primary purpose is educational. In some substance abuse treatment programs, the Twelve Steps are integrated into the program and made part of earned treatment privileges. Some treatment programs provide random, temporary sponsorship, as discussed in Chapter 6. Often these temporary sponsors are provided by local 12-step fellowships. Their role is to accompany treatment patients to meetings, familiarize them with the format, offer support when the going is rough, and follow up with phone calls to make sure meeting attendance continues. Later, when patients have found a fellowship that best fulfills their needs, they make contact with their own personal sponsor.

NA holds Bridge Meetings that are part of their public information service. These meetings are conducted in many settings to introduce newcomers to the 12-step philosophy in general and to NA in particular and to encourage attendance at community meetings.

Within treatment facilities, it has become more common for counselors and staff members to have firsthand knowledge of alcoholism and addiction through family members or to be in recovery themselves (Staub and Kent 1973). The understanding of alcoholism and addiction as a disease has removed much of the moral stigma from open acknowledgment of substance abuse problems. Many people in active recovery, especially those experienced in the 12-step programs, realize the importance of sharing the struggle toward recovery. The acknowledgment of substance abuse problems and recovery by prominent public figures contributes to the acceptance and support of individuals successfully confronting their addictions. On the other hand, public disclosure can occur too soon, ultimately proving detrimental to the individual; hence the emphasis on anonymity.

Al-Anon and Alateen meetings are held at many substance abuse treatment centers, correctional facilities, and other residential programs. Many members of 12-step programs acknowledge that they grew up in a family dominated by alcoholism or addiction and use Al-Anon or Alateen to help them overcome the legacy of a difficult childhood.

In addition, the AA magazine *Grapevine* is considered by many members as a "meeting in print," offering an opportunity to share alcoholism issues with prospective members and interested professionals. Readers have reported its usefulness for relapse prevention, finding it a useful vehicle for bridging the gap between treatment programs and community 12-step meetings (Alcoholics Anonymous 1990–1991).

Halfway Houses

Halfway houses, quarterway houses, and other residential facilities provide a transition between addiction treatment programs and complete return to the community. Most individuals enter halfway houses from inpatient treatment facilities. During their stay, which could vary from a few months to more than a year, they often continue their interrupted schooling through participation in a general equivalency diploma (GED) program or job training. Counselors work with residents to find an apprenticeship program or an entry-level job. These important skills for re-entry to the community are accompanied by multiple opportunities to attend 12-step meetings. Meetings are often held several times a week in-house and are sometimes open to the community. Former residents frequently return for meetings and the opportunity to socialize without the temptation of drugs and alcohol. Halfway houses are usually located near public transportation and often have vans available to transport residents to other meetings. Twelve-step literature is read aloud before and during meals, and references to 12-step philosophy are often part of the general conversation.

Oxford Houses are a recent arrival on the recovery scene, modeled on the principles of AA and NA. Each house is established as an alcohol- and drug-free environment to support recovery and reentry into the community. As with the 12-step meetings, each Oxford House is run democratically with no paid staff, which encourages alcoholics and addicts to help themselves by helping one another. Each resident pays a share of the rent, making the houses self-supporting and promoting stable employment for the residents. The length of stay is indeterminate; residents themselves decide when they are ready to move on to independent living. Although no 12-step meetings are held at Oxford Houses, members attend an average of six AA or NA meetings per week. Attendance at AA or NA meetings is not formally required because these are programs of attraction, not promotion, but it is strongly encouraged. As residents routinely attend meetings, newcomers to Oxford Houses gradually join them and begin to understand and appreciate the role of the meetings in lasting recovery. When setting up a new Oxford House, individual AA or NA members may offer assistance through such activities as helping collect household items for the residence (Molloy 1990; O'Neill 1990), with the understanding that this constitutes no endorsement or affiliation by the 12-step fellowship.

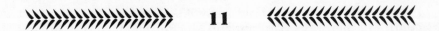

11

The Criminal Justice System

- Drug Use and Crime
- DWI Programs
- Juvenile Justice Programs

The National Institute of Justice (NIJ) estimates that in 1989, 1 out of every 46 adults in the United States was under some type of correctional supervision. As of the end of 1989, 2,520,479 adults were on probation, 456,797 were on parole, and 1,105,607 were incarcerated in prisons or jails (Bureau of Justice Statistics 1991). NIJ's Drug Use Forecasting (DUF) system, which measures drug use by those arrested on serious criminal charges, reported in the third quarter of 1991 that 23% to 74% of the male booked arrestees who volunteered tested positive for at least one drug, depending on the city where the testing took place (National Institute of Justice 1992). These figures indicate that a conservative estimate of drug use (not including alcohol) in the criminal justice system approaches 3 million adult users of illicit drugs. Adding individuals with serious alcohol problems, but without concomitant drug problems, would increase the number significantly. Addicted offenders in the criminal justice system are often the hardcore, chemically dependent individuals with the poorest prognoses. They are the ones who create the greatest social costs, and they are also the most likely to be afflicted with multiple social handicaps and to be in greatest need of help to recover control of their lives (DuPont and MacKenzie 1993; DuPont and Wish 1992).

Given the enormity of the problem of substance abuse in the criminal justice system, the potential for 12-step programs to have a significant impact on the drug and alcohol problem is obvious. The crowded conditions of correctional facilities have resulted in a massive strain on correctional budgets, making it crucial to implement low-cost, effective programs that help offenders abstain from drug and alcohol use. Twelve-step programs offer the advantages of being low cost and replicable. Holding community meetings within minimum-security facilities encourages offenders to maintain a commitment to the program after their release.

Within jails and prisons, AA and NA fellowships provide an opportunity for offenders to participate in a socially acceptable, rehabilitative activity (Wexler et al. 1988). Many inmates admit to attending their first 12-step meetings primarily as an alternative to sitting in a jail cell. San Quentin prison in California is implementing an innovative drug treatment program that includes participation in a 12-step program by inmates interested in achieving a drug-free life-style (Enright 1991). AA publishes guidelines for setting up meetings in prisons and jails and includes information to encourage the newly released individual to maintain ties to 12-step programs in the community (Alcoholics Anonymous 1990c). One of the most compelling arguments for this approach is the role of the peer group in the addict's or alcoholic's behavior. Offenders, by becoming involved in a 12-step group, are surrounded by a new group of peers committed not just to abstinence but to other prosocial behaviors as well. Finding a permanent sponsor forges a connection to a positive role model. Following release from incarceration, the ultimate goal beyond abstinence is involvement in the Twelfth Step—that is, reaching out to other offenders to enhance one's own recovery.

A high correlation exists between alcohol and other drug use and crime (Bureau of Justice Statistics 1989). Probation and parole programs are increasingly mandating abstinence from drug and alcohol use as a condition of release, often enforcing the policy with routine (and random) urine drug tests. Encouraging participation in 12-step programs supports court orders to remain drug-free and provides a new network of prosocial contacts in the community. Familiarizing parole and probation officers with the fellowships and providing them with lists of meeting times and places facilitates access to the programs. As part of the Twelfth Step, which encourages carrying the message to other addicts and alcoholics, recruiting temporary or regular sponsors from the community provides a more tangible link to the 12-step fellowships.

The judicial system is making increasing use of AA meetings as part of DWI (or DUI) sanctions. Jurisdictions vary considerably in the sanctions imposed on convicted drunk drivers. For instance, in some California counties, a first or second DUI conviction (depending on the driver's blood alcohol level at the time of arrest) results in a fine, a period of up to 1 year's probation, mandatory attendance at three consecutive evening sessions of DUI School, and mandatory attendance at AA meetings (usually one to three times a week, with encouragement to attend more).

One problem inherent in routinely ordering DWI and DUI offenders to attend AA meetings is that a person arrested for such a driving violation may not necessarily be an alcoholic or even a problem drinker. Although it is certainly appropriate for even the onetime inebriated driver to be arrested, it may be less appropriate for this person to be channeled into a series of AA meetings. The individual may feel out of place and resentful of this placement, and the supportive nature of the fellowship may suffer from vocal manifestations of such reluctance. Even if the attendees are not overtly negative in their attitude toward being at the meeting, in certain large cities, droves of newcomers who are unaware of how meetings work may have a deleterious effect on a meeting's dynamics.

This problem is substantially reduced in jurisdictions that use evaluations and referral mechanisms similar to those used by employee assistance programs (EAPs) in the workplace and student assistance programs (SAPs) in schools. Some criminal justice agencies evaluate each arrested driver and make appropriate and personalized treatment plans. For those who are referred to 12-step meetings, special educational programs introducing them to 12-step programs are conducted. The use of institutional meetings within the criminal justice agency educates the arrested driver to the 12-step fellowships. Linking the arrested driver with a temporary sponsor is another excellent way to bridge the gap between the DWI program and 12-step fellowships.

An ongoing controversy surrounding mandatory attendance is the perceived religious overtones of the 12-step fellowships. Although, as discussed earlier, the emphasis of the recovery groups is on spirituality and not on any organized religion, individuals who reject formalized religion often do not understand the difference and resist an introduction to the 12-step programs. Self-help addiction groups exist that do not build on a spiritual base and may be considered as an alternative for individuals uncomfortable with the concept of a Higher Power. Examples of these groups include Secular Organizations for Sobriety, Methods of Moderation (formerly American Atheist Addiction Recovery Groups), and Rational Recovery Systems (White and Madara 1992).

At least one study has shown that offenders convicted of DWI charges whose probation officers recommended AA meetings stayed with the meetings longer than voluntary participants. Although there was a high attrition rate following the first meeting, after 6 months a significantly greater percentage of probationers remained active in AA meetings (Rosenberg and Liftik 1976).

Detention centers are frequently an offender's (and especially a juvenile's) first experience with the correctional system. The length of stay at a juvenile detention center varies considerably from one jurisdiction to another (Office of Juvenile Justice and Delinquency Prevention 1991). More juvenile detention programs are instituting pretrial drug testing, which gives the counselor information about drug use to present to the offender immediately and to use for case management (DuPont et al. 1990). Case management presents an ideal opportunity to introduce 12-step meetings as one component in a plan to help offenders reach and maintain drug-free status.

Twelve-step programs have been implemented successfully in some juvenile detention programs. In Washington State, AA and NA have been brought into the correctional institutions with considerable enthusiasm on both sides. Although it is usually preferable to link participants with meetings in the community, that approach is often prohibitive for security reasons in correctional settings. The state of Washington works closely with AA and NA to bring open 12-step meetings into the institutions. After an initial period of resistance to having AA and NA meetings brought in, open communication between treatment staff and 12-step volunteers has resulted in a program "owned" by AA and NA and firmly supported by the correctional treatment staff. The content of the meetings is not modified in any way by the institution. Instead, the institutional treatment program incorporates education on the Twelve Steps into the overall recovery process (D. Brenna, personal communication, March 1991).

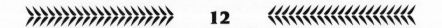

12

Educational Institutions

- Student Assistance Programs
- Colleges and Universities
- Medical Education

Secondary Schools and Universities

In the United States in 1988, there were 20,758 public secondary schools with a total enrollment of 16,200,000 and 3,587 schools of higher education with a total enrollment of 12,800,000 (Bureau of the Census 1990).

The onset of alcohol and other drug use often takes place during the teenage years, a time most people are in school. For Americans, schools traditionally have been the major social institutions to convey not only the three "R"s but also cultural values and community identity. The epidemic of drug and alcohol abuse that began in schools more than 20 years ago has had profound negative effects on families, communities, and schools. Today, schools play an important role not only in helping youth avoid and (if necessary) overcome addiction, but also in helping the families of students recognize and intervene in problems of addiction in both students and parents. The 12-step revolution can play an important role in this effort.

As families become more fragmented through divorce, outside employment by both parents, and greater distance from extended family, the involvement of other social institutions has become more important. In times past, churches and neighborhoods filled needs that families were unable to meet. Today, especially in urban areas, many of these support systems are missing. Schools have come to play an increasingly important social role in many communities. From before- and after-school day care to parenting classes for pregnant high school students, schools are asked to accept many of the tasks that once were assumed to be the family's responsibility. Teachers frequently are called on to assume the role of social worker; guidance counselors, formerly restricted to high schools, are now working with elementary school students.

Although there is disagreement about the current role of the schools—that is, whether it is solely to impart knowledge or to provide a more holistic function—there is little question that alcohol and drug abuse must be addressed. Increasingly, the patchwork of programs and individual efforts is becoming systematized into guidance programs that involve support personnel throughout the school system. One such effort, which was begun on a small scale, is the student assistance program (SAP).

SAPs are patterned after employee assistance programs (EAPs), which are described in Chapter 13. SAPs are usually high school programs that provide support to students with chemical dependence and other behavioral or emotional problems. A student may self-refer or may be referred by a faculty or staff member who identifies a potential problem the student is experiencing (McGovern and DuPont 1991; Office of Substance Abuse Prevention 1988).

Although other components are present in an SAP, support groups in the form of AA, NA, Al-Anon, and Alateen often make up an important part of an SAP program. Issues of confidentiality may prevent teachers and administrators from directly identifying and referring students to 12-step programs. Instead, guidance counselors as part of an SAP team can encourage participation in AA or Alateen meetings by making literature available, posting meeting times and locations, and encouraging students to speak with a peer already involved in one of the 12-step programs. In some cases, the meetings are modified to complement the developmental stages of adolescents. Meetings usually are held at a time and place convenient to student schedules and transportation constraints, and anonymity is assured.

The 1990 Al-Anon/Alateen Membership Survey revealed that 11% of all Alateen meetings are held in schools, up from 1% in 1987 (Al-Anon 1991). Al-Anon members, through their Cooperating with the Professional Community (CPC) committees, reach out to faculty and students at the elementary and secondary school levels. Alateen meetings have an Al-Anon member who serves as the group's sponsor, but the teens themselves conduct the meeting. Typically the Al-Anon member is not a parent of one of the teens present. These 12-step programs convey an essential message to this age group—that they are not "in this alone," and that there is support and understanding from others who share the same issues of coping and recovery. At a vulnerable stage for high-risk youth, such affirmation and fellowship can mean the difference between long-term struggle and successful recovery (Al-Anon 1969).

Alcoholics Anonymous has begun to reach out to faculty members of elementary schools and high schools by offering the services of CPC committee members. Panels of AA members have gone to schools to discuss AA and to share personal experiences (Alcoholics Anonymous 1989a). This education of educators is yet another way of enhancing the referral process.

In recent years, 12-step fellowships increasingly are holding meetings on university campuses. Removed from family and community support systems, college students, many of whom are on their own for the first time, find themselves in a new environment with totally different expectations. They are vulnerable to the easy availability of alcohol and other drugs on or near campus. Removed from customary behavioral boundaries, students frequently succumb to social pressure. The probability of recidivism for those who have undergone substance abuse treatment is increased. Students who choose not to use alcohol or drugs, includ-

ing those who have been through treatment, often face ostracism
and self-imposed isolation from social activities. Usually desperate
for drug-free activities and social support groups, these students
can be plagued by anxiety and depression. Similar consequences
can be found among faculty and staff who do not conform to per-
missive philosophies of alcohol and other drug use that promote
"collegial congeniality" or, in some instances, myths of "mind-
expanding experiences."

When AA, NA, and other 12-step groups meet on or near college campuses, they offer a drug-free support system and social
network for both students and faculty. They also encourage early
recognition of substance abuse problems and encourage recovery
early in the addictive process. Unfortunately, many campuses do
not have 12-step programs or do not openly publicize meetings.
Denial of drug and excessive alcohol use on college campuses by
administrators has limited publicity about drug-free efforts, including 12-step meetings. Institutions of higher education have op-
erated on the premise that promoting drug-free activities and
support services acknowledges that alcohol and other drug problems are prevalent on campus, which may result in a negative public image for the institution.

In many communities, religious organizations commonly
sponsor 12-step programs; campus ministries often sponsor meetings for the college community. However, meetings can be hard to
find. On some campuses, meetings are advertised in student news-
papers, although these ads are cryptic if one is unfamiliar with the
host, "Bill W." Occasionally, referrals are made through student
health services, counseling centers, or wellness programs.

Tacit acceptance of alcohol use on many college campuses
presents formidable obstacles. By playing to the national ambiva-
lence of society toward drinking, emphasis is placed on programs
that teach students to behave "responsibly" about alcohol rather
than promoting abstinence and respect for the legal drinking age
of 21. For those who have completed substance abuse treatment,
or those on a collision course with addiction, "responsible use" can
portend disaster.

The 1989 Drug Act Amendments have played an important role in bringing about changes in policies and attitudes in institutions of higher education. Although some colleges and universities have merely enacted policies that technically conform to U.S. Department of Education guidelines, other schools have questioned the presence of alcohol on campuses at all. A few colleges have banned all forms of alcohol for all ages, creating "dry" campuses. With the application of the "drug-free workplace" to academe, higher education has been forced to address drug use within the campus community. In an unprecedented speech before the Intercollegiate Forum at San Diego in 1990, Robin Wilson, president of California State University at Chico, stated that the "ubiquitous use of booze" (p. 14) lay behind most of the serious problems facing campuses and their surrounding communities—date rape, suicide, fist fights outside bars, homicides, arson, drug abuse, drownings, and automobile accidents ("Better times at Chico State" 1990).

Twelve-step programs and other drug-free activities on campuses promote drug-free environments with visible social and support group activities that emphasize the unacceptability of alcohol and other drug use. They also promote respect for self and others and responsibility for personal behavior. There is a great need to increase the availability of these programs on campuses across the country.

Medical Schools

A great potential exists for educating medical doctors more fully in the disease of alcoholism and drug addiction and in the 12-step programs. In 1987, according to the U.S. Department of Education, 122 medical schools conferred 15,620 medical degrees on graduates. This number represents a significant potential source of referrals to 12-step fellowships.

Educating future medical professionals in the 12-step recovery philosophy is compatible with medical and psychiatric treatment of substance abuse. The medical community is increasingly recognizing that recovery, rather than abstinence alone, is the appropriate goal for drug and alcohol treatment. Recovery involves an improved quality of life that is achieved most often through regular participation in a 12-step program (Chappel et al. 1990; Hanlon 1985).

Alcoholics Anonymous works with medical schools through its CPC committees. AA reaches out to the medical community by inviting medical students to attend open AA meetings, by arranging for AA representatives to speak to medical classes, and by "sponsoring" individual students (Alcoholics Anonymous 1989a). Medical faculty who are themselves members of AA have initiated efforts to have the disease of alcoholism covered more adequately in the medical curriculum. Similar activities are also sponsored by Al-Anon to inform the medical community about the effect of alcohol use on the families and friends of alcoholics.

Several medical schools have begun to include exposure to the 12-step philosophy in their curricula. For example, Georgetown University School of Medicine requires that all first-year medical students attend a 12-step meeting. This requirement exposes prospective physicians to the 12-step philosophy of recovery and provides an opportunity for the students themselves to get help if needed during a stressful educational process.

The University of Nevada School of Medicine introduced substance abuse education into its medical school curriculum in 1974. In 1987, a clinical training program was begun with the aid of a recovering medical student and incorporated into the third-year psychiatric clerkship. The program's focus familiarizes physicians with the 12-step programs to support patients in recovery. The basic component of the experience is to attend four or more 12-step meetings alone and another set of meetings with a recovery guide. Recovery guides—volunteers from AA and NA—meet with individual medical students to provide information and share reactions to the program (Chappel et al. 1990).

The Betty Ford Center, an alcohol and drug addiction treatment facility in Rancho Mirage, California, began a medical student summer school program in 1988. Medical students from around the country, mostly first-year students, attend the primarily experiential weeklong session. An important component of the multidisciplinary treatment approach is involvement in AA. One of the greatest achievements of the medical student program is the students' dramatic change in attitude toward addictive disease and the realization that those with addictions can get well (Vance 1992).

Medical school curricula, as ever, remain full and demanding. Yet the scope of the disease problems of alcoholism and drug addiction is so devastating, in both depth and breadth, to our nation's health that room must be found in those curricula to more adequately address these problems. No single therapeutic measure is as effective for these issues of addiction as the 12-step fellowships. No student should graduate from medical school without being aware of them and how to "prescribe" them.

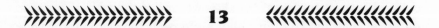 **13**

Religious Organizations

- Role of the Clergy
- Denominational Networks
- Catholic and Jewish Recovery Organizations

Because Alcoholics Anonymous grew out of the Oxford Group, founded by a clergyman after the turn of the century, the link between the religious community and the 12-step programs is especially significant. As we discussed earlier, many essential elements of AA are taken from the practices and philosophies of early Christianity.

The 12-step fellowships and organized religion share a unique relationship. Some individuals see an irony in that organized religion was initially responsible for the moral stigma attached to drunkenness (and later to any alcohol consumption outside religious ceremonies) and the fact that today churches are the primary location of 12-step meetings in many communities.

Spirituality as espoused by 12-step fellowships can conflict with institutionalized religion on both ends of the spectrum. Atheists frequently express concern with the religious overtones that spirituality and "God as we understood Him" implies. Use of the Lord's Prayer is often alien to non-Christians. Religion and spirituality can become confused in the minds of individuals

101

first encountering 12-step fellowships.

People from traditional religious backgrounds may have difficulty with the concept of "God as we understood Him" for very different reasons. To them, such a phrase is too vague to provide guidance for an alcoholic or anyone else. Expecting people to define their own Higher Power seems incomprehensible, inappropriate, and even offensive to some religious individuals.

As with professionals in other fields, the role of the clergy is important to the referral process. Especially in small communities and rural areas, troubled individuals frequently seek help from a member of the clergy. Clergy can play a crucial role in referring parishioners to 12-step programs, providing them with assurance that this path is appropriate, effective, and compatible with their faith. When provincial mores create a problem, the assurance of anonymity in 12-step programs may encourage participation. Clergy need to familiarize themselves with individual community fellowships to ensure that their recommendations are appropriate to the individual and to the group. Clergy are more easily able to follow up a referral because of their ongoing relationship with parishioners. Not only are they able to find out if the person actually attended the meeting and made a satisfactory connection, but they can provide parallel pastoral support during the recovery process.

Congregational policy can increase accessibility to 12-step fellowships. Houses of worship often provide space for 12-step meetings at nominal cost, but they can give the programs greater visibility by listing the meetings among the activities and opportunities available to the community. Outreach to the community is a priority of many congregations. Reaching out to a group of individuals in need of understanding and emotional support is very much in the spirit of service of many religious groups.

Ministering to those in need takes many forms. Providing guidance and referral to 12-step programs to someone with alcoholism or drug addiction can save a body as well as a soul. Welcoming an Alateen group may promote the kind of spiritual healing and growth that a youth ministry program might want to foster (Madara and Peterson 1987).

Seminary students preparing for the clergy should be familiarized with 12-step fellowships as part of their training in counseling. As with medical or educational professionals, they should be given adequate preparation and background before attending meetings, and they should be encouraged to consider ways to incorporate meeting referrals into their counseling options. AA has worked with seminaries by offering to "sponsor" students, taking them to open meetings and answering their questions about alcoholism (Alcoholics Anonymous 1989a). Even more influential may be continuing education programs for clergy once they are in the field. As with many professions, specific skills and knowledge are not always recognized as important during the training process. Once ministers, priests, rabbis, and other members of the clergy become involved with congregations, it becomes apparent how many lives are touched by alcoholism and addiction. Families in crisis frequently turn to their spiritual advisers for help. Holding conferences for clergy on the addiction process and on how to make effective referral to treatment, including the 12-step fellowships, can enhance introductions to the fellowships.

Increasingly, members of the clergy are attending workshops on addictions and becoming familiar with alcoholism as a disease. Many know that AA and the other 12-step programs "work" to help the individual who is addicted achieve abstinence and promote long-term recovery from both drugs and alcohol. Despite that progress, the view of alcoholism and addiction as sinful dies hard in the religious community. Education needs to focus on eliminating moralism and guilt. Clergy still have difficulty understanding denial as a symptom of the disease and not as a moral failure or an example of human willfulness.

Several religious denominations have telephone networks for clergy to contact a central phone number and be connected with a person in a nearby parish or community who is affiliated with a 12-step fellowship. Religious groups with a strong central organization can more easily establish such a network, but it also is possible for autonomous congregations to set up similar plans. AA encourages contact by mailing invitations for information to clergy and following up with telephone calls (Alcoholics Anonymous 1989a).

The National Interfaith Network on Alcohol and Drugs (NINAD) is one example of an organization seeking to address alcohol and drug abuse issues through faith communities. NINAD encourages creative measures to form a link between religious communities and those with alcohol and drug abuse problems. One innovative program in Texas called Project ADEPT (Alcohol and Drug Education in the Parishes of Texas) is funded by a grant from the Texas Commission on Alcohol and Drug Abuse and administered by the Texas Conference of Churches. This project trains clergy and congregational teams from several major denominations in three communities to minister to individuals affected by drug and alcohol abuse. The focus of the ministry is a "bridge" class that discusses passages from the Bible and relates the message to the person's progression through the 12-step pathway to recovery. This approach of connecting a personal and corporate faith journey with the 12-step road to recovery offers a unique opportunity to merge spiritual growth with emotional and physical recovery (Merrill 1990). The National Episcopal Coalition on Alcohol and Drugs (NECAD) is an example of a denominational group addressing the problems of alcohol and drug abuse. NECAD encourages the diocese to form Commissions on Alcoholism, provides networking information for these groups, and addresses questions such as "Should alcoholics ingest the wine at the Eucharist?"

Over 20 years ago, an Episcopal clergyman in recovery founded the Recovering Alcoholic Clergy Association (RACA). Membership in the group is restricted to Episcopal clergy, although clergy in other denominations are now developing their own fellowships. RACA provides a place where clergy can enjoy relaxed fellowship while working on the personal and professional problems of alcoholism and drug abuse.

The religious communities of Atlanta offer several programs addressing the problems of alcohol and drug abuse through introductions to 12-step fellowships. The Episcopal Diocese of Atlanta sponsors spirituality retreats offering fun, fellowship, and workshops on the 12-step recovery programs. These retreats are run by church workers who have received CHART (Community Health and Recovery Teams) training. CHART teams are trained to provide support to individuals seeking help for an alcohol or drug problem. They have the resources to connect the addict or alcoholic with a 12-step member who can provide information on the 12-step programs, accompany the person to meetings, and offer support during the early recovery process.

The churches in Atlanta have also set up more than 20 halfway houses called Metro Atlanta Recovery Residences that offer extended care for recovering alcoholics and addicts. The residents of each house are linked with a church in the neighborhood that sponsors an AA group with church members in attendance. The church includes residents in its activities and programs, providing a supportive community during the recovery process. Churches in other communities support similar halfway houses and group homes for recovering alcoholics and addicts.

An interdenominational Alcohol and Drug Awareness Sunday is held on the Sunday before Thanksgiving in Atlanta in the Catholic, Episcopal, and Presbyterian churches, as well as others. The service includes substance abuse awareness information, sharing of personal experiences, and education about the 12-step programs.

A Catholic organization known as the Calix Society describes itself as an "extension of AA." Founded by five alcoholics in 1947, its role is not to supplant, but rather to augment, the 12-step program. "Calix," the Latin word for "chalice," was chosen to signify that "the cup that sanctifies" was exchanged for "the cup that stupefies." Members are expected to remain active in AA. Calix meetings usually follow a Mass and are structured to enhance sobriety through spiritual growth and a return to a faith that had been neglected (Calix Society, undated; Fox 1992).

The Jewish Alcoholics, Chemically Dependent Persons and Significant Others (JACS) Foundation was founded in 1980 to address the issue of alcoholism and chemical dependency in the Jewish population. JACS is not a 12-step program; rather, it acts as a resource center for recovery information. An important component of the JACS program is the semiannual retreat for recovering individuals and family members involving spiritual renewal and participation in AA and Al-Anon meetings and discussions. JACS firmly supports the tenets of AA and encourages alcoholic and addicted members of the Jewish faith to look beyond the unfamiliar prayers to the recovery potential of the program. The Twelve Steps of AA and the concept of a Higher Power are compatible with the beliefs of Judaism. Synagogues are encouraged to welcome AA and NA meetings (Robertson 1988; Twerski 1986; White and Madara 1992). The JACS Foundation is a striking example of an organization that builds much-needed bridges to 12-step programs of recovery.

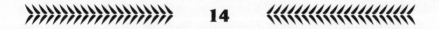

The Workplace

- Alcohol and Drug Use Policies
- Employee Assistance Programs

As of January 1991, there were 116,922,000 people employed in the United States. From corporate CEOs to fast-food workers, most adult Americans spend part of most days at work. A large proportion of this work force is touched by alcoholism and addiction, either personally or through a family member or friend. The economic well-being of our country is affected by alcohol and drug use through accidents, carelessness, increased absenteeism, and inattention. Although drug testing is beginning to address the issue of drug use that carries over into the workplace, the problems that drugs and alcohol pose go much deeper than the results of a drug test.

The workplace is a common place for addiction to be identified because of the adverse effect on work performance. It is also an excellent location for making introductions to 12-step programs and for the development of family-based prevention opportunities. Modern workplace substance abuse prevention programs are comprehensive responses to the problems of alcoholism and addiction. In addition to employee assistance programs (EAPs), comprehensive workplace programs include

establishing written policies for the abuse of alcohol and other
drugs and defining the consequences for violations of these policies. Workplaces are often linked to formal addiction treatment
through employer-sponsored health insurance. Workplace initiatives today increasingly include supervisor training to identify alco-
hol- and other drug-related problems and to help supervisors
make more effective referrals to evaluation, often to EAPs (which
are explained in further detail in the next section). Drug and alcohol testing is often a component of a workplace prevention program (APT Foundation Task Force 1988; Dogoloff and Angarola
1985; DuPont 1989, 1990c; Walsh and Gust 1989). Additional information on workplace prevention programs can be obtained
from the National Institute on Drug Abuse (NIDA), listed in the
Appendix.

Workplace drug prevention programs include provisions for
self-reporting drug problems. The typical result is referral to an
inpatient addiction treatment program or an outpatient treatment
program. However, recovery is much more than abstaining from
drugs or alcohol. Life-style changes are also necessary. Support
from others who have "been there" can enhance the recovery process and sustain long-term abstinence. Although some drug treatment programs stress 12-step aftercare, making the connection to
an appropriate meeting is sometimes difficult. Having 12-step programs available on-site is a convenient method of making the meetings accessible. Often these meetings are BYOL (bring your own
lunch) and held at noon in a conference room (Alcoholics Anonymous 1990b).

In the workplace, 12-step programs present a model of hope,
emphasizing optimism and practicality in overcoming the disease
of alcoholism or drug addiction rather than seeing addiction in
moralistic and fatalistic terms. Industry recognizes the 12-step approach to recovery as being very effective in altering unacceptable
behavior of employees in the workplace by leading them to recovery and improved job performance (Thorne 1989).

The role of 12-step fellowships in the workplace is still being
defined. Employers are becoming more attuned to the needs of

workers and are beginning to offer such support services as child care, fitness opportunities, and smoking cessation groups. An openness exists in mutual-aid groups that enhances participation of employees and contributes to worker satisfaction. However, the holding of "anonymous" groups that address addictions and recovery does present the problem of confidentiality. In an environment where individuals encounter one another on a day-to-day basis and may be colleagues within an office, the issues of revealing and discussing debilitating problems with co-workers are complex (Dory 1990).

One response to this concern is to recognize the limitations placed on a workplace situation and work within those constraints. Using a sponsor or an individual within the group to share especially sensitive topics can be helpful, as the confidentiality of an individual can be more easily assured. An objective opinion can often help determine whether it is appropriate to share information with the larger group. During the preliminary remarks before the start of most fellowship meetings, a statement regarding confidentiality is read. A statement specifically addressing the trust that is inherent in the sharing of experiences at meetings may be helpful as an additional reminder (Kathleen W. 1989).

Employee Assistance Programs

Alcoholics Anonymous has a strong relationship with the EAP movement in the United States. In 1940, a recovering alcoholic and AA member became the first industrial counselor specifically assigned to work with alcoholics and addicts. A subsidiary of the DuPont Corporation established a case-finding and referral system that concentrated on late-stage alcoholics; this system was heavily dependent on the experience of AA. In recent years, there has been a steady growth of occupational alcoholism programs. Since the 1960s, these programs have increasingly included a focus on other drugs in addition to alcohol.

Although the Sixth Tradition of Alcoholics Anonymous enjoins the fellowship from active association with "any related facility or outside enterprise," the influence of its members continues to be manifest in workplace-related activities. Through their public information services, members of AA have made presentations to corporate management, worked with alcoholic colleagues, and set an example of recovery in the workplace (Alcoholics Anonymous 1989a).

More education on the problems associated with the drug-free workplace is needed. Too many misconceptions are attached to the processes of addiction and recovery. Although the recognition of alcoholism and drug addiction as diseases should have removed the moral stigma, it has not, and the process of recovery and the road to abstinence are still fraught with pain for many people. Access to 12-step fellowships can alleviate much of the distress, but sometimes getting the access itself is not an easy process. Worksites need to make available meeting places for 12-step meetings. Anonymity may be a concern in the workplace, but it can be made less of one if the meetings are open or if EAP programs firmly support participation.

Within some professions, mutual-aid groups or networks have been developed to address specific alcohol and other drug issues for that profession or institution (e.g., International Doctors in AA, Academics in Recovery Together, Dentists Concerned for Dentists, and Psychologists Helping Psychologists).

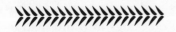 **15**

Recommendations to Increase Access to 12-Step Programs

- Meeting the Needs of Alcoholics and Addicts
- Women
- Minority Populations
- Rural Communities
- Community Education
- Education of Professionals
- Relevant 12-Step Literature

Despite the considerable impact of the 12-step programs on individuals and social institutions, there are numerous gaps in access to 12-step programs and the services provided by them. The following recommendations, listed with comments and suggestions, address these needs.

1. Fellowships should meet the needs of the alcoholic, addict, or family member, rather than those of the institution.

Social institutions are becoming more aware of the wisdom of this statement. The institution should facilitate use of the 12-step fellowships but make no effort to interfere with or to direct the fellowships themselves. As we discussed earlier, more and more alcohol and drug treatment facilities and correctional institutions are bringing community 12-step meetings into the institution intact, offering space for meetings in return for inclusion of patients and inmates in them. Whenever feasible, groups of patients or inmates are escorted to community meetings. Treatment and corrections personnel are becoming increasingly aware that those introduced to the 12-step meetings are more likely to continue attending them if the experience is directly transferable. Formal linkages between institutions and community 12-step meetings encourage active members to work with patients or inmates as part of their Twelfth Step work, often becoming sponsors or temporary sponsors.

2. Twelve-step groups need to meet the needs of alcoholic and addicted women.

Women alcoholics differ from men alcoholics in several significant ways. According to one study, more of them are divorced, have other psychiatric disorders, tend to drink alone, feel a greater social stigma attached to their drinking, and have a poorer prognosis for sobriety (Priyadarsini 1986). Other studies, however, have reached different conclusions about recovery outcome. Differences between men and women in terms of drinking behavior, consumption patterns, mortality rates, and physiological differences make interpreting treatment outcome data a complicated business (Hill 1986). A recent British study revealed that, in most studies, there was no difference in treatment outcome based on gender (Jarvis 1992). As can be seen, much of the evidence is mixed and complex.

Interactions among group members often reflect gender differences in participants. Men tend to initiate discussion and dominate interactions. In the presence of men, women often take a more passive role and are less likely to participate. Many women function according to traditional social roles and are less likely to discuss feelings of shame or weakness in past behavior in the presence of men (Priyadarsini 1986).

A potential problem for younger women in 12-step programs is to be approached by older men and to become involved in an inappropriate relationship. Although the roles certainly can be reversed, newly recovering young women tend to be vulnerable to the attention of men who take advantage of the atmosphere of trust and intimacy at 12-step meetings. Such a situation is known as thirteenth stepping (Gregson and Summers 1992).

On the positive side, women who attend mixed groups are frequently able to engage in healthy social relationships with recovering men in a relatively controlled environment. In fact, AA reports that the percentage of women participants in North America has risen from 22% to 34% in the last 22 years (Covington 1991).

Women sometimes feel excluded by the choice of language and the somewhat paternalistic tone of the early 12-step literature, and they are sometimes less comfortable with the idea of powerlessness espoused in the Twelve Steps (Kirkpatrick 1986). However, Stephanie Covington (1991), in her writing about women and mutual-aid groups, explains the paradox of AA in the following way:

> When people get to AA it is because they are in fact powerless to bring about desired feelings or to accomplish their goals without using alcohol. Admitting powerlessness can be a comforting and empowering act and it is a premise of AA that deserves elaboration. The paradox is that admitting where you are powerless in life actually empowers you. It allows you to be in touch with personal power, areas of your life where you do have power and control.
>
> Admission to powerlessness over alcohol permits the identification of times when choices can be made and things can be changed. (p. 89)

AA literature that was written a couple of generations ago contains what many now label as sexist language. To widen the appeal of AA literature, suggestions have been made to rewrite the "Big Book" (1976) and other materials in more inclusive language. Other increasingly obvious moves, such as providing child care during meetings, would increase accessibility for some women (and some men) to attend meetings. In addition, some AA and other 12-step groups have been formed exclusively for women.

3. Twelve-step groups need to have a greater relevance to minority communities.

There is a diversity of opinion among treatment experts and recovering members of 12-step fellowships concerning the adequacy of the current approach to minority communities. Some people believe that minority groups have long felt excluded from 12-step programs and that some ethnic communities regard the meetings as primarily white, middle-class enclaves (Rawson 1990). These members of the drug treatment community believe that ethnic experiences enhance the special meaning of recovery for a specific ethnic group. Others feel equally strongly that ethnic distinctions tend to disappear among fellowship members when the universal issues of alcoholism and addiction are addressed. Most members of ethnic minority groups recognize the acceptance and sharing among members as the primary strength of the 12-step program. The focus is on the shared experience of addiction rather than on personal identity factors. As one minority group member stated, "We're all different. Our illness is our alikeness. It gives us a common bond" (Alcoholics Anonymous 1991).

Beginning with AA, the 12-step programs have created an entirely new culture, with its own language, rituals, and literature. This culture promotes bonding and intimacy, but it can also make the program hard to penetrate. A "we-they" dichotomy is easy to create, making those on the outside perceive themselves as unwelcome. It is therefore not surprising that those who see themselves as outside the mainstream culture have difficulty accepting 12-step recovery.

Many people who are ethnic minorities receive alcohol and other drug treatment through the public sector. Until recently, publicly funded substance abuse treatment programs did not use 12-step programs as extensively as did private providers. With people of color representing a minority in the general population, and with fewer being exposed to the 12-step programs through drug abuse treatment, there have been fewer "messengers" to carry the word about 12-step fellowship.

Within the African American community especially, the recovery model is very different from the recovery model in the white middle-class community. In the latter community, an intervention is usually precipitated by family, friends, and co-workers of the impaired individual. This planned intervention then leads to appropriate treatment. In the African American community, an intervention crisis often is spurred by the criminal justice system. Courts frequently make referrals to public-sector treatment alternatives, and recovery is often maintained through churches with largely African American congregations that are primarily fundamentalist in approach (P. Bell, personal communication, May 1991).

Issues of cultural relevancy are being addressed by AA. Subcommittees have been formed to identify specific cultural groups for the purpose of overcoming barriers to participation. One AA pamphlet is entitled "Do You Think You're Different?" (1993c). Another booklet contains recovery stories featuring American Indians (Alcoholics Anonymous 1991). Most of the AA literature is now available in Spanish, and an AA Hispanic region has been formed in California.

Alcoholics Anonymous drafted suggestions for outreach to minorities in the *Public Information/Cooperation With the Professional Community (PI/CPC) Bulletin* (Alcoholics Anonymous 1989c). These suggestions include training PI/CPC members of varying backgrounds to carry the message to social institutions, providing media material for dissemination to publications and to radio and television stations that target minority interests, contacting professionals who work primarily in minority neighborhoods, and holding PI/CPC meetings in ethnic communities (Alcoholics Anonymous 1989a). AA also has participated in several conferences with national organizations that address the specific issues of minority populations (Alcoholics Anonymous 1991).

4. Special attention needs to be paid to the important role of 12-step meetings in rural areas.

The greatest diversity and selection of 12-step meetings occurs in urban areas where there is sufficient population to support these groups. Individuals seeking 12-step meetings can find them almost around the clock. There are meetings targeting young people, nonsmokers, gay men and lesbians, women, Spanish-speaking people, or Jewish people. They can be found on bus lines and in workplaces. In addition to long-established groups, there are myriad drug-specific groups.

Rural areas present a very different situation for 12-step groups. There is generally a limited availability of meetings, in terms of both time and distance. Communities may have just one meeting per week that is usually heterogeneous in composition. If an individual does not feel comfortable with a particular group, there are fewer alternatives available. Given the fact that most drug and alcohol treatment programs are located in or near urban areas, individuals in rural areas often find that 12-step programs provide vital support, both as an alternative to primary treatment and as aftercare.

Important issues confront individuals seeking help from a 12-step program in a rural area. Anonymity is a concern in small communities where everyone tends to know everyone else. The high school band leader, the minister's spouse, and the local barber may all encounter one another at an AA meeting. Cars parked at the community center or church social hall are easily recognized. Meetings may be scattered widely over a geographical area. The suggestion to attend 90 meetings in 90 days may be impractical if distances of 50 miles or more separate the meeting locations. There are no easy solutions to these problems. However, effective introductions to 12-step programs may include suggestions for ride sharing among members and heightened sensitivity to anonymity issues. The use of telephone and computer networks among fellowship members can help make individuals feel part of the group process. Residents of rural areas can be encouraged to be creative in their efforts to overcome the limitations of distance and scattered population (Talley 1990).

5. More community education is needed.

A New Public Health 1990 Conference was held in April 1990 in Los Angeles to educate representatives of public and private health care organizations about self-help groups, including 12-step fellowships. The 3-day conference, where former U.S. Surgeon General C. Everett Koop gave the keynote address, drew more than 1,500 participants ("Self-help fair brings self-helpers and public health professionals together" 1990).

Alcoholics Anonymous held a Share-A-Day in New York City attended by 4,000 people, half of whom were from minority groups. This open AA meeting familiarized the public with the fellowship (F. Riessman, personal communication, September 1990).

6. Professionals need to build "half the bridge" to 12-step fellowships.

Many people dealing with their own or someone else's chemical dependence seek the help of a professional. Often these professionals are health care workers, but they may also be attorneys or experts in other fields associated with the problems of chemical dependence. These professionals need to build "half the bridge" to 12-step programs. That means using the 10 techniques discussed in Chapter 8 to strengthen the referral process. AA, NA, and Al-Anon can help by "sponsoring" professionals.

7. Literature needs to be available in diverse languages and at various reading levels.

AA's "Big Book" (1976) is written at a seventh-grade reading level (Mills 1989). Large-print editions of some of the literature are available for those with impaired vision. An illustrated version of the Twelve Steps with a primary school reading level has been approved for use in the criminal justice system. A videotape of Chapter Five of the "Big Book" is available in American Sign

Language for the hearing impaired. Audiocassettes of the main
books of AA are available for those with reading difficulties or
visual impairment. Braille versions of the "Big Book" and Twelve
Steps and Twelve Traditions have also been published. The technique AA uses to adapt material to a foreign language is to trans-
late the "Big Book" into a specific language, and then gradually
replace the stories with those from that indigenous culture. This
translation and adaptation technique has been used with Spanish and various Latino cultures, and the process is now under
way in Russian. Other 12-step fellowships need to follow the lead
of AA to make their programs more widely accessible in increasingly diverse communities worldwide.

Section III

Research Agenda

The natural history of alcoholism and drug addiction is a relatively new area of scientific inquiry. Although addiction to alcohol and other drugs, once established in an individual's life, tends to be persistent, many drug abusers stop drug use for varying lengths of time. The recent evidence of a downturn in drug and alcohol use indicators supports the view that many Americans have decreased their use of alcohol and other drugs in recent years. The role of various interventions in stopping drug and alcohol use and in achieving what is increasingly called "recovery" remains a matter of intense research interest. A generation of follow-up studies begun in the 1970s at the National Institute on Drug Abuse (NIDA) and the National Institute on Alcohol Abuse and Alcoholism (NIAAA) has shown that treatment works, less well than some had hoped but far better than many had expected (National Institute on Drug Abuse 1989a; Office of National Drug Control Policy 1990; U.S. Department of Health and Human Services 1990a, 1990b; Wesson et al. 1986). One-year abstinence rates following inpatient alcoholism treatment vary from 50% to 90% depending on patient characteristics, motivation, and continuing participation in aftercare, including 12-step programs (Hoffman and Miller 1992; Kammeier and Laundergan 1977; Miller and Gold 1992;

Thurstin et al. 1987). Treatment outcome was similar for middle-class inpatient and outpatient treatment participants (Alterman et al. 1991). One of the most robust findings of follow-up studies is that the longer an alcoholic or addict stays active in substance abuse treatment, the better the long-term outcome (De Leon 1990; Stimmel 1991).

With respect to participation in 12-step programs, it is now widely acknowledged that these recovery programs do not work for those who try them and drop out, and that lasting recovery is often a prolonged process that frequently includes one or more relapses along the road to recovery. The earlier generation of studies from NIDA and NIAAA failed to collect data on attendance at 12-step meetings in the study samples, so they offer little help in identifying the role of 12-step programs in achieving recovery. The researchers who conducted these studies did not include data on 12-step attendance, because the use of these programs by clients in publicly funded treatment was limited until the 1980s. The current follow-up studies of both NIDA and NIAAA are assessing the role of 12-step programs in recovery rates. One of the most encouraging outcomes of drug and alcohol treatment is the direct correlation between the number of 12-step meetings attended over time and the likelihood of the study subject maintaining recovery (Sheeren 1988). The Seventh Special Report to the U.S. Congress on Alcohol and Health from the Secretary of Health and Human Services (U.S. Department of Health and Human Services 1990c) states, "Investigators suggested that AA could be particularly valuable as a means of aftercare." On the other hand, research also demonstrates that many people who have been treated for chemical dependency are able to establish and maintain recovery without attending 12-step meetings.

Future research must define more precisely (and in prospective studies) who stays with the 12-step programs and who does not, what bridges to the 12-step programs are most successful, and what can be done to improve the introduction process in the future. These questions are the focus of this book.

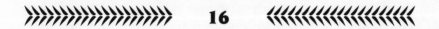

Published Research Findings

- Twelve-Step Attendance and Recovery
- Characteristics of 12-Step Participants

Although Alcoholics Anonymous and other 12-step recovery programs are generally recognized by the addiction community, by the professional substance abuse treatment community, and increasingly by the general public as a valuable part of the recovery process of alcoholism and addiction, published research into the mechanisms involved is sparse. The Seventh Special Report to the U.S. Congress on Alcohol and Health from the Secretary of Health and Human Services (U.S. Department of Health and Human Services 1990c) credits AA for a useful role in promoting and maintaining abstinence.

Descriptive studies show a positive relationship between 12-step attendance and successful treatment outcome for many recovering alcoholics and addicts (Anderson and Gilbert 1989; Giannetti 1981; Hoffmann et al. 1983; Rawson 1990; Thurstin et al. 1987; Westermeyer 1989). A recent study by Hoffman and Miller (1992) supports the positive correlation between AA attendance and continuing abstinence following inpatient or outpatient treatment. This study found that about 70% of individuals who completed inpatient or outpatient treatment based on a 12-step model and attended regular AA meetings maintained abstinence after 1 year.

Exactly which components of the 12-step programs contribute to the recovery process is not yet clear. It is also not clear which participants are most affected. One theory is that participation in a support group enhances chances for recovery (Hoffmann et al. 1983; Powell 1987). The Hoffmann research team determined that there is a high correlation between weekly attendance at AA meetings and long-term abstinence during aftercare following inpatient substance abuse treatment. During the course of treatment, patients were introduced to the principles of AA and worked through the first three to five steps of AA as part of the program. Follow-up results suggest that alcoholics going to AA meetings are twice as likely to maintain sobriety 6 months following treatment as those who do not. Another interesting outcome was that patients either tended to follow the recommendations of the treatment staff to attend 12-step meetings regularly or chose to ignore the advice completely and not attend meetings at all. Very few chose the middle ground of desultory attendance. Another study supported systematic encouragement of alcoholics to attend and to increase participation in 12-step meetings in the community (Sisson and Mallams 1981).

A study conducted in the State of New York considered AA members' perception of the importance of the 12-step fellowship in maintaining recovery as compared to an outpatient treatment program. At the conclusion of the study, participants were surveyed to ascertain the relative importance of AA participation and outpatient counseling on maintaining sobriety. Those with greater than the median days of sobriety attached significantly greater importance to their affiliation with AA. The results reinforce the assumption that AA plays an important role in long-term recovery (Williams et al. 1986).

Another study conducted in England that compared abstainers, controlled drinkers, and relapsers using AA as an abstinence program concluded, "Those patients who have been exposed to a total abstinence model, and who have attempted abstinence and have been moderately successful, have the highest chance of becoming long-term abstainers" (Elal-Lawrence et al. 1986, p. 45). A similar study concluded that the likelihood of relapse correlated strongly with the level of involvement in AA. The areas of commitment to the fellowship that were most important were a strong relationship with a sponsor and active 12-step work (Sheeren 1988).

A study of physicians impaired by alcohol and other drug use was conducted by Galanter and colleagues (1990), who found that combining traditional psychotherapy with 12-step programs provided effective treatment and constructive aftercare. Within the treatment program, a special 12-step group was formed to provide a bridge to community 12-step meetings. Physicians who sustained stable recovery attributed their success to affiliation with the 12-step programs, reporting that "intensity of commitment to AA was a significant predictor of perceived benefit" (Galanter et al. 1990, p. 66).

An attempt was made to identify an "alcoholic personality" by establishing Minnesota Multiphasic Personality Inventory (MMPI; Hathaway and McKinley 1970) profiles of successful participants in AA programs and those who chose not to attend 12-step meetings. This study established that there was little personality difference between alcoholics who attended AA meetings regularly and those who did not. Attendance at AA meetings does not appear to be predictable based on specific personality traits (Thurstin et al. 1986).

Twelve-step fellowships may not be appropriate for everyone, at least in the traditional format that exists in many locations. Some studies have shown that AA is least successful among those from lower socioeconomic levels and with individuals displaying major psychiatric disorders (Hoffmann et al. 1983; Smith 1986).

Although these studies shed some light on the efficacy of 12-step programs, they leave many unanswered questions, especially those addressing the introductory process. Chapter 17 outlines research issues for future consideration.

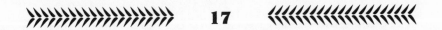

Research Issues for 12-Step Introductions

- Established Identity of 12-Step Programs
- Need to Study and Improve Referral Process
- Characteristics of 12-Step Programs
- Impact of Simultaneous Professional Treatment
- Attitudes and Beliefs of Attendees
- Institutional Support
- Introductory Mechanisms

In relation to their size and impact, there has been comparatively little study of 12-step programs. Twelve-step programs have neither sought nor accepted research and have little to gain from being the focus of research. These programs, unlike all other drug and alcohol treatment programs, have no need to prove their efficacy as a means to obtain funding, to receive official licenses to operate, to gain public support, or to attract clients. Twelve-step programs see themselves as needing no modification based on research. Current methods are accepted on the basis of experience, and enough participants are confident of the outcome to make change based on research unnecessary and quite possibly counterproductive. The usual objectives of evaluative study include

1. Assessing the efficacy (worth) of a particular intervention;
2. Learning the mechanisms involved; and/or
3. Understanding how to make that intervention more effective.

From the perspective of the 12-step programs, social science research is likely to create problems and offer no effective help. The needed expertise is contained within the program itself.

The growth of AA, NA, and the other 12-step fellowships does not reflect a political or a funding decision; instead, it reflects millions of personal choices being made every day. This dynamic historical process offers an opportunity to learn, scientifically, from this "experiment of nature." We do not have to assume a priori that one or the other approach to referral is better. Instead, we can study the process and learn with the best interest of the referred alcoholic, addict, or family member as our guide. Although the objectives of research and the autonomy of the 12-step programs are not questioned, other issues are worthy of study that do not presume an invasive approach into or a change in 12-step programming. These issues permit the 12-step programs to reach more people by promoting wider professional and public support for the 12-step movement. These approaches, which we have discussed in this book, focus on the introductory process, not on the 12-step fellowships themselves.

How can the referral process be improved to increase the likelihood that individuals in need of support connect with the 12-step fellowships? What factors in referral increase the likelihood of long-term abstinence and other prosocial objectives? Descriptive studies are useful in understanding differences in the characteristics of onetime, sporadic, and regular meeting attendees. Understanding demography and background as well as referral source, community support systems, alcohol and drug use history, and optimism or pessimism about achieving abstinence may provide suggestions about characteristics of individuals who may need more or less support in achieving regular 12-step attendance. Specifically, factors that encourage greater use of 12-step programs need to be studied through

1. An understanding of who attends and who does not attend 12-step meetings following referral;
2. Knowledge of issues that gain support from health professionals and formal and informal social institutions;
3. Exploration of alternative referral mechanisms; and
4. Acknowledgment of other social issues affecting the referral process and its likelihood of success.

What are the characteristics of people who attend or do not attend 12-step meetings after referral?   A number of important issues invite descriptive study. The physical needs, psychological conditions, and emotional states of individuals with addictions can be assessed as they are in the process of deciding whether or not to participate in a 12-step program. This type of study could be established in a consortium of treatment centers.

It would be important to know the stage of addiction at which a new recruit encounters a 12-step group and is most receptive to its message. A study could assess the relative efficacy of involvement in 12-step meetings early in the addictive career versus later involvement. Efficacy is defined as both attendance and retention in 12-step meetings and achievement of abstinence and other prosocial goals. It would be helpful to know more about who attends 12-step meetings only after a long history of denial and who attends with relatively new problems of addiction.

A study needs to be conducted of alcoholics and addicts (matched for age and primary drug of abuse) who attend 12-step meetings only (never in formal treatment) with those who attend formal treatment only (never in 12-step meetings). Such a study would involve an examination of demographic and background characteristics as we have outlined here. Most important, the study would examine attitudes and beliefs about 12-step programs and professionally run treatment programs. The study would attempt to clarify concerns and misgivings about both 12-step and professional treatment in an effort to allow both to be properly accessible.

An unknown number of individuals elect or are encouraged to affiliate with both 12-step and professional alcohol and other drug treatment. The extent of voluntary, simultaneous participation in both professional treatment and 12-step programs needs to be explored. Clients need to be surveyed to find out their reasons for dual attendance, to learn how they see the two methods of service delivery as complementing each other, and to ascertain whether they see problems in the coordination or integration of those services.

Another question concerns the attitudes and beliefs of potential recruits regarding "typical" 12-step members. What preconceived opinions do newcomers bring with them to meetings that have implications for referral? Issues such as the perceived religious orientation of the meetings or the idea that participants are very different from newcomers need to be explored. It would be useful to discover how those initial thoughts are reinforced or supplanted by subsequent personal experience.

Identifying the differences between participants and nonparticipants in the 12-step fellowships would be valuable. Rather than looking only at personality differences, it would be useful also to explore such trait differences as feelings of hopelessness or lack of control, feelings of empowerment, feelings of isolation, and levels of self-esteem.

Attitudes and beliefs about 12-step programs among minority group members, women, young people, and elderly people are important to examine. We need to determine the preconceptions and misconceptions that exist among populations that feel excluded from participation in 12-step programs.

The controversy regarding the perceived religious overtones of the 12-step programs suggests a study of individuals making a choice between 12-step fellowships and other self-help groups. What is the likelihood of success in terms of stopping use of alcohol and other drugs?

Finally, it would be informative to learn why some people in long-term recovery eventually quit attending 12-step meetings. Do the programs become self-limiting in their ability to sustain participation, and is the tendency to move on to other avenues of growth seen as a positive step in the recovery process?

What are the issues that support referrals to 12-step programs from health professionals and social institutions?
Just as we have insufficient descriptive data regarding attendees of 12-step programs, we need more data on 12-step program use by community agencies. More exact surveys are needed on the extent to which 12-step programs are employed by

1. Substance abuse treatment programs;
2. Medical professionals;
3. The criminal justice system;
4. The workplace;
5. Religious organizations; and
6. Colleges and other educational institutions.

Within each organization surveyed, information collected would include the total number of clients seen by each administrative structure or service program in relation to its total population, length of time the program has been in place, and staffing patterns. Most important, we need to assess the extent of referral from social agencies to 12-step programs, including the number of clients referred monthly or annually, the method of making referrals, the types of clients referred, the point in the client's career at which referral is initiated, the follow-up strategy to determine attendance, and the staff involved in making and supporting the referrals.

Professionals in the field of addictions treatment have a long-standing interest in the criminal justice population. Correctional institutions are especially receptive to 12-step meetings. Little research is available about 12-step groups in criminal justice programs, including institutional attitudes toward 12-step programs

and the extent to which the meetings are encouraged and supported by criminal justice agencies such as prisons and probation
or parole programs. Demographic and background characteristics
and attitudes about 12-step meetings among attendees and non-
attendees of 12-step programs in criminal justice settings should be
studied. A particular concern is the relationship of 12-step programs to prosocial life goals, including abstinence from alcohol
and other drug use, productive employment, and cessation of
crime.

Additional study is needed to assess the efficacy of different
strategies in referral for achieving regular and long-term attendance at 12-step meetings. An effective liaison between formal
treatment and 12-step fellowships provides aftercare programming
and complements the strength of formal treatment with the effectiveness of potentially lifelong aftercare. In this instance, studies
could compare the use of on-site 12-step meetings by formal treatment programs to active referral by treatment programs to off-site
12-step meetings (e.g., assignment of a temporary sponsor to es-
cort a client to the 12-step site and follow up to see if the client went
to the meetings) to passive referral (e.g., a suggestion that the client attend a 12-step meeting).

**What introductory mechanisms encourage attendance and
retention in 12-step meetings?**   Surveys of attitudes and beliefs about 12-step programs are needed among

1. Drug and alcohol abuse treatment providers;
2. Private health care practitioners;
3. EAP staff;
4. Correctional and criminal justice administrators and service
    providers; and
5. School health officials.

A survey of this type would determine their knowledge of and
receptivity to the process of referral to 12-step fellowships.

Beyond the level of descriptive study, quasi-experimental research can be employed to examine the effects of various referral strategies on meeting attendance and maintenance of alcohol- and drug-free status. A study could compare the results of court-mandated referral and voluntary referral on attendance at 12-step meetings and on achievement of prosocial goals. In addition to comparing mandated to voluntary referral, different methods of referral support need to be determined. Within-group study can explore characteristics of frequent and infrequent attendance within the mandated referral group and (separately) within the voluntary referral group. An important initial task would be to define what constitutes a "voluntary referral," because such referrals usually involve a complex interaction of family, job, friendship, and other pressures leading to self-referral.

Attendance and retention in 12-step programs are useful proxy measures for program efficacy in the same way retention is used as a proxy measure for treatment efficacy by professional drug abuse treatment programs. However, it is not a direct test of efficacy. That outcome would require follow-up in the community to assess drug use, criminal activity, or prosocial achievements at selected intervals postintervention.

Additional research of referral strategies could study motivators to 12-step involvement and retention. Various specific strategies to involve family members in the referral process could be evaluated. Similarly, different sponsor characteristics and different strategies for using sponsors can be evaluated.

Special issues in 12-step referral can also be subjected to study. Attendance and retention rates can be explored in relation to the practices of different 12-step programs, such as the different emphases placed on socialization outside of meetings and on linkages to community groups.

What other social issues should be addressed in the introductory process? The primary purpose of this type of research is to increase the availability and efficacy of interventions to combat alcohol and other drug abuse. In that spirit, studies are suggested to clarify the characteristics of 12-step attendees before and after referral, to understand attitudes and beliefs about 12-step programs among the potential social agents of referral, and to explore the capacity of different referral strategies for achieving attendance and retention in 12-step fellowships.

Epilogue

This book reflects a modest effort to educate social institutions, and the professionals affiliated with them, and to help them improve referral techniques to 12-step programs. This effort recognizes and celebrates the power of the miracle of recovery that is found within these unique programs. Although not proposing invasive research into the 12-step programs themselves, our discussion here calls for a new generation of insight and research into the referral processes that form bridges between social institutions and the 12-step fellowships. This effort can help people all over the world to overcome the diseases of alcoholism and drug addiction.

References

Alcohol, Drug Abuse and Mental Health Administration: National Drug and Alcoholism Treatment Unit Survey 1989: Main Findings Report. Rockville, MD, U.S. Department of Health and Human Services, 1990

Al-Anon: Purpose and Suggestions. New York, Al-Anon Family Group Headquarters, 1969

Al-Anon: Al-Anon Is for Adult Children of Alcoholics. New York, Al-Anon Family Group Headquarters, 1983

Al-Anon: Al-Anon Family Groups. New York, Al-Anon Family Group Headquarters, 1984

Al-Anon: One Day at a Time in Al-Anon. New York, Al-Anon Family Group Headquarters, 1985

Al-Anon: Al-Anon Speaks to You, the Professional. New York, Al-Anon Family Group Headquarters, 1987

Al-Anon: Alateen—Hope for Children of Alcoholics. New York, Al-Anon Family Group Headquarters, 1989

Al-Anon: Al-Anon Faces Alcoholism, 2nd Edition. New York, Al-Anon Family Group Headquarters, 1990a

Al-Anon: . . . In All Our Affairs: Making Crises Work for You. New York, Al-Anon Family Group Headquarters, 1990b

Al-Anon: 1990 Al-Anon/Alateen Membership Survey. New York, Al-Anon Family Group Headquarters, 1991

Al-Anon: Courage to Change. New York, Al-Anon Family Group Headquarters, 1992

Alcoholics Anonymous: Came to Believe. . . . New York, Alcoholics Anonymous World Services, 1973

Alcoholics Anonymous: Living Sober: Some Methods AA Members Have Used for Not Drinking. New York, Alcoholics Anonymous World Services, 1975

Alcoholics Anonymous: Alcoholics Anonymous, 3rd Edition. New York, Alcoholics Anonymous World Services, 1976

Alcoholics Anonymous: Dr. Bob and the Good Oldtimers: A Biography, With Recollections of Early AA in the Midwest. New York, Alcoholics Anonymous World Services, 1980

Alcoholics Anonymous: Cooperation with the Professional Community (CPC). New York, Alcoholics Anonymous World Services, 1989a

Alcoholics Anonymous: The case for Alcoholics Anonymous, in Chemical Dependency: Opposing Viewpoints. Edited by Davis S. San Diego, CA, Greenhaven Press, 1989b

Alcoholics Anonymous: Public Information/Cooperation With the Professional Community Bulletin. New York, Alcoholics Anonymous World Services, Fall 1989c

Alcoholics Anonymous: Alcoholics Anonymous 1989 Membership Survey. New York, Alcoholics Anonymous World Services, 1990a

Alcoholics Anonymous: Where and When. New York, Alcoholics Anonymous World Services, 1990b

Alcoholics Anonymous: AA in Correctional Facilities. New York, Alcoholics Anonymous World Services, 1990c

Alcoholics Anonymous: The AA Grapevine: a meeting in print. New York, Alcoholics Anonymous World Services, Winter 1990–1991

Alcoholics Anonymous: About AA. New York, Alcoholics Anonymous World Services, 1991

Alcoholics Anonymous: The AA Member—Medications and Other Drugs. New York, Alcoholics Anonymous World Services, 1992a

Alcoholics Anonymous: AA in Treatment Facilities. New York, Alcoholics Anonymous World Services, 1992b

Alcoholics Anonymous: Members of the Clergy Ask About Alcoholics Anonymous. New York, Alcoholics Anonymous World Services, 1992c

Alcoholics Anonymous: Questions and Answers on Sponsorship. New York, Alcoholics Anonymous World Services, 1993a

Alcoholics Anonymous: AA as a Resource for the Health Care Professional. New York, Alcoholics Anonymous World Services, 1993b

Alcoholics Anonymous: Do you think you're different? New York, Alcoholics Anonymous World Services, 1993c

Alcoholics Anonymous: 44 Questions? New York, Alcoholics Anonymous World Services, 1993d

Alterman AI, O'Brien CP, McLellan AT: Differential therapeutics for substance abuse, in Clinical Textbook of Addictive Disorders. Edited by Francis RJ, Miller SI. New York, Guilford, 1991, pp 369–390

Anderson JG, Gilbert FS: Communication skills training with alcoholics for improving performance of two of the Alcoholics Anonymous recovery steps. J Stud Alcohol 50(4):361–366, 1989

APT Foundation Task Force: Report on Drug and Alcohol Testing in the Workplace. New Haven, CT, APT Foundation, 1988

Ashery RS: Self-help groups serving drug abusers, in Addicts and Aftercare: Sage Annual Reviews of Drug and Alcohol Abuse. Edited by Brown BS. Beverly Hills, CA, Sage, 1979

Better times at Chico State. Prevention Pipeline 5(4):13–16, Fall 1990

Bureau of the Census: Statistical Abstract of the United States. Washington, DC, U.S. Department of Commerce, 1990

Bureau of Justice Statistics: Correctional Populations in the United States, 1988. Washington, DC, U.S. Department of Justice, 1991

Bureau of Justice Statistics: Drug Use and Crime: Special Report. Washington, DC, U.S. Department of Justice, 1989

Calix Society: How It Works—Spiritually. Minneapolis, MN, undated

Cermak TL: Evaluating and Treating Adult Children of Alcoholics. Minneapolis, MN, Johnson Institute, 1990

Chappel JN: Spirituality is not necessarily religion: a commentary on "divine intervention and the treatment of chemical dependency." Substance Abuse 2:481–483, 1990

Chappel JN: The use of Alcoholics Anonymous and Narcotics Anonymous by the physician in treating drug and alcohol addiction, in Comprehensive Handbook of Drug and Alcohol Addiction. Edited by Miller N. New York, Marcel Dekker, 1991, pp 1079–1088

Chappel JN, Veach TL, Klein B: Teaching medical students to utilize 12-step programs. J Subst Abuse 11(3):142–150, 1990

Covington SS: Sororities of helping and healing: women and mutual help groups, in Alcohol and Drugs Are Women's Issues, Vol 1. Edited by Roth P. Metuchen, NJ, Women's Action Alliance and Scarecrow Press, 1991, pp 85–92

De Leon G: Treatment strategies, in Handbook of Drug Control in the United States. Edited by Inciardi JA. Westport, CT, Greenwood Press, 1990, pp 115–138

Dogoloff LI, Angarola RT: Urine Testing in the Workplace. Rockville, MD, American Council for Drug Education, 1985

Dory FJ: Self-help groups at the workplace: investment in employees' well-being. Self-Helper 5(3):2, 1990

DuPont RL: Getting Unhooked: A Guide to the Twelve-Step Programs. Rockville, MD, DuPont Associates, 1989

DuPont RL: A clinician's view of the epidemiology of anxiety disorders. Paper presented at the Psychiatric Times' 3rd Annual U.S. Psychiatric Congress, San Diego, CA, December 1990a

DuPont RL: Benzodiazepines and chemical dependence: clinical guidelines. Paper presented to the Conference on Practical Clinical Management: Drug Abuse Education for the Primary Case Physician, Baltimore, MD, October 1990b

DuPont RL: Medicines and drug testing in the workplace. J Psychoactive Drugs 22:451–459, 1990c

DuPont RL, MacKenzie D: Narcotics and drug abuse: an unforeseen tidal wave, in The President's Crime Commission: 25 Years Later (ACJS/Anderson Monograph Series). Edited by Conley JA. Cincinnati, OH, Anderson Publishing Company (in press)

DuPont RL, McGovern JP: Co-dependence: a new diagnosis, parts I and II, in Directions in Psychiatry, Vol 11, Lessons 9 and 10. Edited by Flach F. New York, Hatherleigh, 1991a, pp 1–8

DuPont RL, McGovern JP: The growing impact of the children of alcoholics movement on medicine: a revolution in our midst, in Children of Chemically Dependent Parents: Multiperspectives from the Cutting Edge. Edited by Rivinus TM. New York, Brunner/Mazel, 1991b, pp 313–329

DuPont RL, McGovern JP: Suffering in addiction: alcoholism and drug dependence, in The Hidden Dimension of Illness: Human Suffering. Edited by Starck PL, McGovern JP. New York, National League for Nursing Press, 1992, pp 155–201

DuPont RL, Wish ED: Operation Tripwire revisited, in Drug Abuse: Linking Policy and Research: Annals of the American Academy of Political and Social Science. Edited by Wish ED, Lambert RD, Heston AW. Newbury Park, CA, Sage, 1992, pp 91–111

DuPont RL, Saylor KE, Latimer S: Drug testing: taking the guesswork out of detection. Corrections Today 52(5):168–171, 1990

Elal-Lawrence G, Slade PD, Dewey ME: Predictors of outcome type in treated problem drinkers. J Stud Alcohol 47(1):41–47, 1986

Enright J: San Quentin plans innovative drug program: correction news. California Department of Corrections 4(9):4, March 1991

Ferguson T: Running a self-help group by computer. Medical Self-Care Magazine, November/December 1987, p 80

Fox B: Prayer, sacraments, and sobriety. New Covenant, December 1992, pp 30–31

Galanter M, Talbott D, Gallegos K, et al: Combined Alcoholics Anonymous and professional care for addicted physicians. Am J Psychiatry 147(1):64–68, 1990

Giannetti VJ: Alcoholics Anonymous and the recovering alcoholic: an exploratory study. Am J Drug Alcohol Abuse 8(3):363–369, 1981

Gordis E: Estimating the economic cost of alcohol abuse—a commentary by NIAAA director (Alcohol Alert No 11). Rockville, MD, National Institute on Alcohol Abuse and Alcoholism, U.S. Department of Health and Human Services, January 1991

Gregson D, Summers H: 13th stepping. Professional Counselor 7:33–37, 1992

Hall T: New way to treat alcoholism discards spirituality of AA. New York Times, December 24, 1990, Section A, p 1

Hanlon MJ: A review of the recent literature relating to the training of medical students in alcoholism. J Med Educ 60:618–626, August 1985

Hathaway SR, McKinley JC: Minnesota Multiphasic Personality Inventory, Revised. Minneapolis, MN, University of Minnesota, 1970

Hazelden Foundation: Hazelden Rehabilitation Services. Center City, MN, Hazelden Foundation, 1990

Hazelton D: Signing on to support groups. Focus, October/November 1990, pp 27, 35

Heath AW, Stanton MD: Family therapy, in Clinical Textbook of Addictive Disorders. Edited by Frances RJ, Miller SI. New York, Guilford, 1991, pp 406–430

Hill SY: Physiological effects of alcohol in women, in Women and Alcohol: Health-Related Issues (National Institute on Alcohol Abuse and Alcoholism Research Monograph No 16). Washington, DC, U.S. Department of Health and Human Services, 1986, pp 199–214

Hoffman NG, Miller NS: Treatment outcomes for abstinence-based programs. Psychiatric Annals 22(8):402–408, 1992

Hoffman NG, Harrison PA, Belille CA: Alcoholics Anonymous after treatment: attendance and abstinence. Int J Addict 18(3):311–318, 1983

Holder HD, Blose JO: The reduction of health care costs associated with alcoholism treatment: a 14-year longitudinal study. J Stud Alcohol 53:293–302, 1992

Jarvis TJ: Implications of gender for alcohol treatment research: a quantitative and qualitative review. Br J Addict 87:1249–1261, 1992

Johnson LD, O'Malley PM, Bachman JG: Smoking, drinking, and illicit drug use among American secondary school students, college students, and young adults, 1975–1991 (University of Michigan Institute for Social Research). Rockville, MD, National Institute on Drug Abuse, U.S. Department of Health and Human Services, 1992

Kammeier M, Laundergan JC: The Outcome of Treatment: Patients Admitted to Hazelden in 1975. Center City, MN, Hazelden Foundation, 1977

Kaufman E: Family systems and family therapy of substance abuse: an overview of two decades of research and clinical experience. Int J Addict 20(6,7):897–916, 1985

Khantzian EJ, Mack JE: Alcoholics Anonymous and contemporary psychodynamic theory, in Recent Developments in Alcoholism, Vol 7. Edited by Galanter M. New York, Plenum, 1989

Kirkpatrick J: Turnabout: New Help for the Woman Alcoholic. New York, Bantam Books, 1986

Klerman GL: Treatment of alcoholism [letter]. N Engl J Med 320(6):394–395, 1989

Kurtz E: A.A.: The Story. San Francisco, CA, Harper & Row, 1987

Kurtz E, Ketcham K: The Spirituality of Imperfection: Modern Wisdom From Classic Stories. New York, Bantam Books, 1992

Lamb-Korn J: General Assembly to consider giving drunk drivers options to Alcoholics Anonymous. Baltimore City Paper, February 27, 1991, p A1

Leerhsen C, Lewis SD, Pomper S, et al: Unite and conquer. Newsweek, February 5, 1990, pp 50–55

Leventhal GS, Maton KI, Madara EJ: Systemic organizational support for self-help groups. Am J Orthopsychiatry 58(4):592–603, 1988

Levit KR, Lazenby HC, Cowan CA, et al: National health expenditures, 1990. Health Care Financing Rev 13:29–54, 1991

Levoy G: A place to belong. Health, February 1989, pp 54–57

Lewis DC: Comparison of alcoholism and other medical diseases: an internist's view. Psychiatric Annals 21(5):256–265, 1991

Liskow B, Nickel E, Tunley N: Alcoholics' attitudes toward and experiences with disulfiram. Am J Drug Alcohol Abuse 16(1,2):147–160, 1990a

Liskow B, Powell BJ, Penick EC: Alcoholics and disulfiram. Am J Drug Alcohol Abuse 16(1,2):161–170, 1990b

M Earle: Physician, Heal Thyself! 35 Years of Adventures in Sobriety by an AA "Old-Timer." Minneapolis, MN, CompCare Publishers, 1989

Madara EJ, Peterson BA: Clergy and self-help groups: practical and promising relationships. Pastoral Care 41(3):213–220, 1987

McGovern JP, DuPont RL: Student assistance programs: an important approach to drug abuse prevention. School Health 61:260–264, 1991

McGovern JP, DuPont RL: Co-dependence: the other half of addiction. Houston Medicine 8:5–11, 1992

Merrill T: The Texas experience. National Interfaith Network on Alcohol and Drugs (NINAD) Newsletter (1)3:1, Fall 1990

Milam JR, Ketcham K: Under the Influence: A Guide to the Myths and Realities of Alcoholism. Seattle, WA, Madrona Publishers, 1981

Miller NS (ed): The disease concept of alcoholism and drug addiction, I. Psychiatric Annals 21(4):194–234, 1991a

Miller NS (ed): The disease concept of alcoholism and drug addiction, II. Psychiatric Annals 21(5):256–306, 1991b

Miller NS, Chappel JN: History of the disease concept. Psychiatric Annals 21(4):196–205, 1991

Miller NS, Gold MS: The psychiatrist's role in integrating pharmacological and nonpharmacological treatments for addictive disorders. Psychiatric Annals 22(8):437–440, 1992

Miller NS, Ries R: The role of recovering persons in medical education. Substance Abuse 11(4):237–239, 1990

Mills KR: Readability of Alcoholics Anonymous: how accessible is the "Big Book"? Perceptual and Motor Skills 69:258, 1989

Molloy JP: Self-Run, Self-Supported Houses for More Effective Recovery from Alcohol and Drug Addiction. Washington, DC, Office of Treatment Improvement, U.S. Department of Health and Human Services, 1990

Mooney AJ, Eisenberg A, Eisenberg H: The Recovery Book. New York, Workman Publishing, 1992

Morse RM, Flavin DK: The definition of alcoholism. JAMA 268(8):1012–1014, 1992

Narcotics Anonymous: Sponsorship. Van Nuys, CA, Narcotics Anonymous World Service Office, 1983

Narcotics Anonymous: Narcotics Anonymous, 5th Edition. Van Nuys, CA, Narcotics Anonymous World Service Office, 1988

Narcotics Anonymous: A Guide to Public Information. Van Nuys, CA, Narcotics Anonymous World Service Office, 1989

Narcotics Anonymous: Narcotics Anonymous: A Resource in Your Community. Van Nuys, CA, Narcotics Anonymous World Service Office, 1990

Narcotics Anonymous: A Resource in Your Community. Van Nuys, CA, Narcotics Anonymous World Service Office, January 1991

National Institute on Alcohol Abuse and Alcoholism: Professional Self-Help Groups: Alcohol Health and Research World. Rockville, MD, U.S. Department of Health and Human Services, Fall 1986

National Institute on Alcohol Abuse and Alcoholism: Clinical Training Grants for Faculty Development in Alcohol and Other Drug Use. Rockville, MD, U.S. Department of Health and Human Services, 1991

National Institute on Drug Abuse: September marks celebration of treatment successes (NIDA Notes). Rockville, MD, U.S. Department of Health and Human Services, Spring/Summer 1989a

National Institute on Drug Abuse: National Drug and Alcoholism Treatment Unit Survey, 1987. Rockville, MD, U.S. Department of Health and Human Services, 1989b

National Institute on Drug Abuse: National household survey on drug abuse: population estimates 1991. Washington, DC, U.S. Government Printing Office, 1991

National Institute of Justice: Drug use forecasting: research in brief. Washington, DC, U.S. Department of Justice, June 1992

Nowinski J, Baker S: The Twelve-Step Facilitation Handbook: A Systematic Approach to Early Recovery from Alcoholism and Addiction. New York, Lexington Books, 1992

Nurco DN, Makofsky A: The self-help movement and Narcotics Anonymous. Am J Drug Alcohol Abuse 8(2):139–151, 1981

Nurco DN, Wegner N, Stephenson P, et al: Ex-Addicts' Self-Help Groups. New York, Praeger, 1983

Office of Juvenile Justice and Delinquency Prevention: Children in custody 1989: OJJDP update on statistics. Washington, DC, U.S. Department of Justice, January 1991

Office of National Drug Control Policy: Understanding drug treatment [white paper]. Washington, DC, Executive Office of the President, June 1990

Office of Substance Abuse Prevention: The Fact Is . . . You Can Start a Student Assistance Program. Rockville, MD, U.S. Department of Health and Human Services, 1988

O'Neill J: History of Oxford House, Inc, in Social Model Alcohol Recovery: An Environmental Approach. Edited by Shaw S, Borkman T. Burbank, CA, Bridge Focus, 1990, pp 103–117

Peele S: Diseasing of America. Lexington, MA, Lexington Books, 1989

Peele S: The Truth About Addiction and Recovery. New York, Simon & Schuster, 1991

Powell TJ: Self-Help Organizations and Professional Practice. Silver Spring, MD, National Association of Social Workers, 1987

Priyadarsini S: Gender-role dynamics in an alcohol therapy group, in Alcohol Interventions. Edited by Strug DL, Priyadarsini S, Hyman MM. New York, Haworth, 1986, pp 179–196

Rawson R: Cut the crack: the policymaker's guide to cocaine treatment. Policy Review, Winter 1990, pp 10–19

Regier DA, Farmer ME, Rae DS, et al: Comorbidity of mental disorders with alcohol and other drug abuse. JAMA 264:2511–2518, 1990

Rice DP, Kelman S: Measuring comorbidity and overlap in the hospitalization cost for alcohol and drug abuse and mental illness. Inquiry 26(2):249–260, 1989

Rice DP, Kelman S, Miller LS, et al: The economic costs of alcohol and drug abuse and mental illness: 1985. Washington, DC, U.S. Government Printing Office, 1990

Rice DP, Kelman S, Miller LS: The economic cost of alcohol abuse. Alcohol Health and Research World 15:307–316, 1991

Robertson N: Getting Better: Inside Alcoholics Anonymous. New York, Morrow, 1988

Rosenberg CM, Liftik J: Use of coercion in the outpatient treatment of alcoholism. J Stud Alcohol 37:58–65, 1976

Saylor KE, DuPont RL, Brouillard M: Self-help treatment of anxiety disorders, in Handbook of Anxiety, Vol 4: The Treatment of Anxiety. Edited by Noyes R, Roth M, Burrows GD. Amsterdam, Netherlands, Elsevier, 1990, pp 483–496

Self-help fair brings self-helpers and public health professionals together. Self-Helper 5(3):4, 1990

Seymour RB, Smith DE: Drug Free: A Unique, Positive Approach to Staying Off Alcohol and Other Drugs. New York, Facts On Files Publications, 1987

Sheeren M: The relationship between relapse and involvement in Alcoholics Anonymous. J Stud Alcohol 49(1):104–106, 1988

Siegel WG: Personality, social support, and recidivism among alcoholics. Master's thesis, University of Iowa, 1988

Sisson RW, Mallams JH: The use of systematic encouragement and community access procedures to increase attendance at Alcoholics Anonymous and Al-Anon meetings. Am J Drug Alcohol Abuse 8(3):371–376, 1981

Smith DI: Evaluation of a residential AA program. Int J Addict 21(1):33–49, 1986

Sonnefeld ST, Waldo DR, Lemieus JA, et al: Projections of national health expenditures through the year 2000. Health Care Financing Review 13:1–27, 1991

Staub GE, Kent LM: The Para-Professional in the Treatment of Alcoholism. Springfield, IL, Charles C Thomas, 1973

Stimmel B: Effective treatment for substance abuse: defining the issues. J Addict Dis 11(2):1–4, 1991

Talley E: Is somebody out there? self-help groups in rural areas. Self-Helper 6(1):6, 1990

Thorne CL: Development of an Employee Assistance Program at Washington Metropolitan Area Transit Authority, in Workplace Drug Abuse Policy. Edited by Walsh JM, Gust SW. Rockville, MD, National Institute on Drug Abuse, 1989, pp 89–96

Thurstin AH, Alfano AM, Sherer M: Pretreatment MMPI profiles of AA members and nonmembers. J Stud Alcohol 47(6):468–471, 1986

Thurstin AH, Alfano AM, Nerviano VJ: The efficacy of AA attendance for aftercare of inpatient alcoholics: some follow-up data. Int J Addict 22(11):1083–1090, 1987

Twerski AJ: The Truth About Chemical Dependency and Jews. Aliquippa, PA, Gateway Rehabilitation Center Publications, 1986

U.S. Department of Health and Human Services: Confronting alcohol abuse and dependence: treatment research fortified the front lines. ADAMHA News 16(1):1–2, 1990a

U.S. Department of Health and Human Services: Dr. Goodwin and other agency drug treatment experts brief key Senate staff. ADAMHA News 16(3):2, 1990b

U.S. Department of Health and Human Services: Seventh special report to the U.S. Congress on alcohol and health from the Secretary of Health and Human Services. Rockville, MD, National Institute on Alcohol Abuse and Alcoholism, 1990c

Vance A: It's a question of attitude as much as one of skills—The Betty Ford Center Medical Student Summer Program. Paper presented at the 36th International Congress on Alcohol and Drug Dependence, Glasgow, Scotland, August 1992

W Kathleen: A forum response: on confidentiality. Self-Helper 4(2):7–8, 1989

Walsh JM, Gust SW (eds): Workplace Drug Abuse Policy: National Institute on Drug Abuse Office of Workplace Initiatives. Washington, DC, U.S. Department of Health and Human Services, 1989

Wasserman H, Danforth HE: The Human Bond: Support Groups and Mutual Aid. New York, Spring Publishing, 1988

Wesson DR, Havassy BE, Smith DE: Theories of relapse and recovery and their implications for drug abuse treatment, in Relapse and Recovery in Drug Abuse (NIDA Research Monograph 72). Edited by Tims FM, Leukefeld CG. Rockville, MD, National Institute on Drug Abuse, 1986, pp 5–19

Westermeyer J: Nontreatment factors affecting treatment outcome in substance abuse. Am J Drug Alcohol Abuse 15(1):13–29, 1989

Wexler HK, Lipton DS, Johnson BD: A criminal justice system strategy for treating cocaine-heroin abusing offenders in custody. Washington, DC, National Institute of Justice, U.S. Department of Justice, 1988

White BJ, Madara EJ (eds): The Self-Help Sourcebook, 4th Edition. Denville, NJ, American Self-Help Clearinghouse, St. Clares-Riverside Medical Center, 1992

Williams JF: Current challenges in substance abuse education. Substance Abuse 11(4):240–243, 1990

Williams JM, Stout JK, Erickson L: Comparison of the importance of Alcoholics Anonymous and outpatient counseling to maintenance of sobriety among alcohol abusers. Psychol Rep 58:803–806, 1986

Woititz JG: Adult Children of Alcoholics. Deerfield Beach, FL, Health Communications Inc., 1990

Zweben JE: Counseling issues in methadone maintenance treatment. J Psychoactive Drugs 23(2):177–190, 1991

Appendix

Adult Children of Alcoholics
  World Service Organization
P.O. Box 3216
Torrance, CA 90510
(310) 534-1815

Al-Anon Family Group Headquarters, Inc.
P.O. Box 862—Midtown Station
New York, NY 10018-0862
(212) 302-7240

Alcoholics Anonymous World Services, Inc.
(General Service Office)
Box 459
Grand Central Station
New York, NY 10163
(212) 870-3400

American Self-Help Clearinghouse
St. Clares-Riverside Medical Center
Denville, NJ 07834
(201) 625-7101

American Society of Addiction Medicine (ASAM)
5225 Wisconsin Avenue, N.W., #409
Washington, DC 20015
(202) 244-8948

Center for Substance Abuse Treatment (CSAT)
Substance Abuse and Mental Health
  Services Administration (SAMHSA)
5600 Fishers Lane
Rockville, MD 20857
(301) 443-5052

Hazelden Educational Materials
  Customer Service
15251 Pleasant Valley Road
P.O. Box 176
Center City, MN 55012
(800) 328-9000

JACS (Jewish Alcoholics, Chemically Dependent
  Persons and Significant Others) Foundation
426 West 58th Street
New York, NY 10019
(212) 397-4197

Narcotics Anonymous World Service Office
P.O. Box 9999
Van Nuys, CA 91409
(818) 780-3951

National Clearinghouse for Alcohol and
  Drug Information (NCADI)
P.O. Box 2345
Rockville, MD 20847-2345
(301) 468-2600
(800) 729-6686
(800) 487-4889 (TDD)

National Council on Alcoholism and
  Drug Dependence (NCADD)
12 West 21st Street
New York, NY 10010
(212) 206-6770
or
1511 K Street, N.W., Suite 926
Washington, DC 20005
(202) 737-8122 or (800) NCA-CALL

National Institute on Alcohol Abuse and
  Alcoholism (NIAAA)
5600 Fishers Lane
Rockville, MD 20857
(301) 443-3860

National Institute on Drug Abuse (NIDA)
Division of Workplace Programs (SAMHSA)
5600 Fishers Lane
Rockville, MD 20857
(301) 443-4513

National Self-Help Clearinghouse
25 West 43rd Street, Room 620
New York, NY 10036
(212) 642-2944

Women for Sobriety
P.O. Box 618
Quakertown, PA 18951-0618
(800) 333-1606

Index

*Page numbers printed in **boldface** type refer to tables.*